D1377835

PRAISE FOR DAVID NICO AND *DIET DIAGNOSIS*...

Nico's enthusiasm for sharing the Healthnut way—a lifestyle guided by informed choices that enable physical and spiritual vitality—shines throughout this comprehensive guide on how to be a thoughtful food consumer. From toxins to fad diets to GMOs to cholesterol, Nico speaks to the hot topics at the edge of nutrition to make his points accessible to all readers interested in addressing health where it starts: on your plate.

—*Michael F. Roizen, MD*
Four-time #1 *New York Times* best-selling author

More than just another weight-loss book, David Nico's *Diet Diagnosis* covers everything from detoxification to intermittent fasting, creating an easy-to-apply roadmap that helps you successfully navigate the ever-changing world of fat loss and optimal health to become your best self. A must read!

—*J. J. Virgin*
New York Times best-selling author, *The Virgin Diet*

When one is ready to make a change and choose life, this information is necessary. David's book can help you in your transition. You can abandon your past and let this book become your life coach on the journey to better health.

—*Bernie Siegel, MD*
New York Times best-selling author, *The Art of Healing* and
A Book of Miracles

What a fantastic book! David Nico has written one of the most comprehensive yet practical and easy-to-follow books on healthy living that I've ever read. A primer on wellness and the food industry, a multifaceted life plan, a summary of the best research on diet and nutrition—this book has everything you need to remake yourself into a healthier and fitter you. With Dr. Nico's help, we can all become Healthnuts while enjoying the journey of transformation.

—*Jeff Levin, PhD, MPH*
Professor of Epidemiology and Population Health
Professor of Medical Humanities
Baylor University
Adjunct Professor of Psychiatry and Behavioral Sciences
Duke University School of Medicine
Author, *God, Faith, and Health*

If you are among the millions of Americans who struggle with obesity and are bewildered by the hundreds of diets that have come and gone, let Dr. Healthnut be your guide. This book is based in good science and good sense. Dr. Nico's advice honors the integration of body, mind, and spirit, without which food doesn't nourish and diets don't work.

—*Larry Dossey, MD*
Former chief-of-staff, Medical City Dallas Hospital
New York Times best-selling author

At age ninety-five, and in excellent health, I may be the senior nutrition educator to wholeheartedly endorse this excellent new book. Dr. Nico shares helpful tips, insightful strategies, and practical approaches that can work for anyone. Although most people struggle with dieting, I believe this book has great potential for helping Americans and others worldwide find a better pathway to health and nutrition. Tell your friends and family members to get this book!

—*Dr. Mary Ruth Swope*
Author, professor, and nutrition education pioneer

I have known David Nico for several years and have found him to be a kindred spirit in the world of health and wellness. He is not content with just quick-fix methods that invariably fail after a time, like many so-called experts are, but he is interested in the holistic, long-term healing of the body, mind, and spirit. His depth of insight into the physiology and biochemistry of our complex bodies and minds are impressive for a non-physician. His understanding of the connection between our physical and spiritual health is vitally important in our world today. And he is able to distill the jargon down into understandable language for the common people seeking answers and hope. Dr. David Nico will be a credible voice in the world of health and wellness for many years to come.

—*Alan W. Gruning, DO, FACOEP*
President, International Center for Health and Wellness
President, Christian Health Ministries and the Southwest Florida Free Pain Clinic

If you are either confused about diets or interested in learning more about the dozens of different diet programs and which one might work best for you, then David Nico's book *Diet Diagnosis* will be a valuable resource. But *Diet Diagnosis* is more than just a survey of different types of diet programs. It discusses a wide range of important topics like GMOs, artificial sweeteners, agricultural toxins, and the underlying causes of obesity, plus a healthy dose of encouragement to find the diet that is right for you.

—*Ross Pelton, "The Natural Pharmacist," RPh, PhD, CCN*
Author, *Drug-Induced Nutrient Depletion Handbook*

Ever feel like you can't believe the news you read about diet and nutrition advice because it is constantly changing and contradictory? If your answer to this question is *yes*, then *Diet Diagnosis* is a must-read for you! David Nico shares cutting-edge knowledge and research in an easy-to-read format. This book is the definitive guide on the what, why, and how of diet and nutrition.

—*Christopher P. Neck, PhD*
Author, *Fit to Lead*

Out of the swarm of advisories that emerge daily on how best to fuel our precious machine, few measure up to stellar status. David Nico's *Diet Diagnosis* reflects his twenty-year experience in extracting the essence of nutritional science. This book is a recipe to live by.

—*Walter Bortz, MD*
Clinical professor, Stanford University Medicine School
Author, *Dare to Be 100*

The choice between healthy living or disease living begins with what you put in your mouth. In *Diet Diagnosis*, David Nico helps his readers move beyond gimmick-based diets, which rarely provide longstanding weight loss, to a personalized lifestyle change that provides lifelong wellness. Wellness requires solutions, and solutions to the obesity epidemic require identification of the contributors to obesity. Dr. Nico identifies some of these contributors, the obstacles to wellness found in obesity, and the misguidance found in the weight-loss industry, and he tackles them head-on to provide real-life Healthnut solutions to healthy living. Read Dr. Nico's book to move from disease living to healthy living.

—Nathan Goodyear, MD, FAARM
Author, *Manboob Nation*

Sometime in the twentieth century, science began accumulating facts upon which to base dietary advice, and a veritable flood of "how to" books have appeared, disappeared, and reappeared in different covers, because the fact is, diet is a major factor in everybody's life and well-being. Many myths and erroneous notions have been promulgated in good faith, occasionally leading to the wrong road. David Nico's book is a comprehensive collection of almost all of the sensible diets available. He also gives important help for determining *your* best choice, with alternatives if it doesn't work out the first time.

—Warren M. Levin, MD, FAAFP (ret.), FACN, FAAEM
Author, *Beyond the Yeast Connection*

Paleo? Vegan? Mediterranean diet? There is so much information (and misinformation) about nutrition in our world! Dr. David Nico's book *Diet Diagnosis* will help you navigate the diet maze and get you on the right track, not only for weight loss but also to meet your health goals and truly nourish your body!

—Dr. Izabella Wentz, PharmD, FASCP
New York Times best-selling author, *Hashimoto's Thyroiditis*

As a practitioner of functional medicine, I am frequently asked, "What is the best diet?" so I am delighted to see *Diet Diagnosis*. It helps you discover your unique plan in a way that is easy to understand and apply. It is a powerhouse book of tips, tactics, and approaches that simply work!

—*Hyla Cass, MD*
Author, *8 Weeks to Vibrant Health*

There is nothing nuts about *Diet Diagnosis* written by David Nico, "Dr. Healthnut"! In fact, it is a spot-on ultimate resource when it comes to navigating the maze and craze of diets and health in our modern day! Bravo—what a fun and engaging read. This is another tool I can give my patients who truly just want to feel amazing.

—*Holly Lucille, ND, RN,*
Naturopathic physician and author

As a life coach, I see many people who have created strategies for career success. But those same people frequently have no plan for success in their health. In *Diet Diagnosis*, David Nico shares clear systems for being as intentional about success in your health as you would expect to be in business. It's not genetics, and it's not luck. It's either having an intentional plan or not.

—*Dan Miller*
New York Times best-selling author, *48 Days to the Work You Love*

Trying to make sense of the jumble of published nutritional programs is a real challenge, especially since many of them seem to conflict. With this comprehensive, practical, and useful book, Dr. Nico has provided a wonderful reference to help guide us through this nutritive maze.

—*Julius Torelli, MD, FACC*
Author, *Beyond Cholesterol*
Consulting editor, *The Inflammation-Free Diet Plan*

"How can I lose weight?" is the wrong question. Or at least not the question we should be asking first. Instead, we should approach our nation's weight problem by asking, "Why am I gaining weight in the first place?" David Nico's book *Diet Diagnosis* will help you understand the "why" of weight gain and then follow that with the "how" of weight loss. You'll finish his book with a clear plan for lasting weight-loss success.

—*Michael A. Smith, MD*
Senior health scientist
Life Extension Foundation, Fort Lauderdale, Florida
Author, *The Supplement Pyramid*

To lose weight and regain your health, you need a lifetime plan. Dr. Nico not only does an excellent job of outlining the maze of different diets out there, but more important, gives you the blueprint to end the diet cycle. Find your *Aha!* Choose your healthnut fans who will inspire you, keep you accountable, and accompany you on your journey to optimal health!

—*Trent Orfanos, MD, FACC, ABIHM*
Cardiologist
Associate Professor of Medicine
Indiana University

Nico is a Healthnut master, and he lives and breathes well-being, which should be the primary goal of health care. His beautiful enthusiasm for your ability to make your own culinary, medical, physical, and spiritual choices can help you eat better, live better and refuel better. Nico helps you take your health into your own hands, where it rightfully belongs, with flavor and with love.

—*John La Puma, MD*
New York Times best-selling author, *ChefMD's Big Book of Culinary Medicine*

This fast-moving book shows you exactly what you can do to lose weight, sleep better and have more energy—all day long!

—*Brian Tracy*
Chairman and CEO, Brian Tracy International

Diet Diagnosis is packed with great information. In this insightful book, Dr. Healthnut breaks away from the one-size-fits-all mentality about healthy diet and lifestyle by exploring a variety of options to help individuals find what works best for them. We all have our own journey, and I believe *Diet Diagnosis* provides the tools to navigate that journey, helping us to make wise decisions toward overall health.

—*Beni Johnson*
Senior pastor, Bethel Church, Redding, California
Author, *The Happy Intercessor*

DIET
DIAGNOSIS

DIET
DIAGNOSIS

DAVID NICO, PHD

WHITAKER
HOUSE

Note: This book is not intended to provide medical advice or to take the place of medical advice and treatment from your personal physician. Neither the publisher nor the author takes any responsibility for any possible consequences from any action taken by any person reading or following the information in this book. If readers are taking prescription medications, they should consult with their physicians and not take themselves off prescribed medicines without the proper supervision of a physician. Always consult your physician or other qualified health care professional before undertaking any change in your physical regimen, whether fasting, diet, medications, or exercise.

DIET DIAGNOSIS:
Navigating the Maze of Health and Nutrition Plans

David Nico
www.drhealthnut.com
www.dietdiagnosis.com
www.davidnico.com

ISBN: 978-1-62911-535-1
eBook ISBN: 978-1-62911-287-9
Printed in the United States of America
© 2015 by David Nico

Whitaker House
1030 Hunt Valley Circle
New Kensington, PA 15068
www.whitakerhouse.com

Library of Congress Cataloging-in-Publication Data (Pending)

1 2 3 4 5 6 7 8 9 10 11   **ш**   22 21 20 19 18 17 16 15

I DEDICATE THIS BOOK TO YOU, MY READERS.
MAY GOD RICHLY BLESS YOU WITH ABUNDANT LIFE. JOHN 10:10

CONTENTS

PART THREE: DR. HEALTHNUT NO-NO'S

PART FIVE: DR. HEALTHNUT ACTION

INTRODUCTION

THE PROBLEM

Do you or someone you love struggle with dieting, weight loss, or just knowing how to eat right? As a passionate advocate for wellness, I have often wondered why health books continue to offer their one-size-fits-all approach to dieting. If you've considered this with me, we're not the only ones. The *U.S. Weight Loss & Diet Control Market* study estimates that out of the approximately 150 million people in the US who are overweight or obese, roughly 90 million are do-it-yourself dieters.[1] And yet, worldwide, it is estimated that at least 2.3 billion adults and children struggle with being overweight or obese.[2] According to the World Health Organization, an unhealthy diet is one of four major global health risk factors that lead to diabetes, cancer, and cardiovascular disease.[3]

If it is so easy to eat right, lose weight, and reduce disease risks, why do so many fail in dieting to achieve a healthy weight for life? Is unhealthy eating the only factor that produces a vicious cycle of life-long disease and weight problems? From diet confusion and environmental stress to genetically modified foods, negative emotions, and other complex health issues, you may be confused about potential solutions to the overweight and obesity crisis—collectively known as "OB." *Diet Diagnosis* will provide you with the tools to overcome OB through effective lifestyle principles that you will incorporate into your daily routine—which naturally leads to the lifetime healthy weight remedy you seek.

This book will teach you how to eat like people who make healthier, eco-friendly, and green choices—the people I consider to be the healthiest on the planet. These *"healthnuts"* really aren't crazy—they just want to eat the right foods for their bodies so that they can be active and disease-free. In fact, the following is the main premise of the book, and it's probably something you've heard many times: *What you put in your mouth ultimately transforms into how you feel and look.*

The problem is, although most of us know we need to eat better, most of us don't know how to incorporate it into our busy lives. This book teaches you how to identify the unique solution that works for your lifestyle. Some of the information you may already know, but you'll learn how to apply it in your unique schedule. Most important, keep in mind that some of the information I discuss is girded by science and other information by my personal experiences and observation. This work is based on my twenty years' experience coaching individuals, leaders, and healthcare professionals, as well as observation of my personal health.

THE SOLUTION

Diet Diagnosis will unveil the specific lifestyle practices to help you achieve the same results healthnuts use to melt unhealthy fat and achieve a lifelong healthy weight. I believe just about everyone can benefit from these principles. You may be a leader of an organization seeking ways to reduce rising health care costs—you will appreciate the healthnut summary points. Or you may be a mom with family members who struggle with their weight—you'll enjoy learning how to create a healthy lifestyle plan. Or you may be an expert in all the diets, but feel they have failed you—you will benefit from a lifelong reference of practical health tips. You may be a viewer of the television shows *The Doctors, Dr. Oz,* or *The Biggest Loser.* You may read popular health magazines, listen to health radio programs, be a member of a wellness facility, or just want to promote health in your company. This book will help you become more knowledgeable about your available food choices so you can help yourself and those you love.

Diet Diagnosis provides an overview of the diet industry by decoding the major diet and lifestyle options. You will also learn the differences between toxic and real foods, practical shopping tips, preparation tools for successful meal planning, and how to develop your own comprehensive lifestyle plan. I'll admit, creating your unique wellness blueprint is not for the faint of heart. If you are willing to put in the effort, I guarantee you will discover a major link to your personal health code.

Diet Diagnosis is divided into five parts.

Part One: Dr. Healthnut World

Part One explains why you intuitively have a desire to live at your ideal weight and the three major causes of OB. Why do you struggle? Contributing to the problem is the plethora of diets that bombard you with contradictory messages about weight loss. In chapter 1, you'll learn the three major causes of OB. Chapter 2 describes some of the diet marketing techniques that keep dieters captive year after year. In chapter 3, you'll also learn how to identify the program that works best for you by introducing you to the *Healthnut Life*.

Part Two: Dr. Healthnut Decode

Part Two helps you decode several diets. Chapter 4 reviews the typical American diet and the three major diets. Chapter 5 discusses the three most popular diets. In chapter 6, you'll discover three specialty diets. You'll also learn why calorie-counting is not necessarily part of successful long-term dieters' lifestyle plans.

Part Three: Dr. Healthnut No-No's

Part Three explains which foods and beverages are most damaging. You'll gain an understanding of the foods that are harmful because they contribute to addictive eating patterns, destroy your metabolism, and prevent you from sustaining a healthy weight. Chapters 7, 8, and 9 inspire you to avoid negative habits by revealing toxic food culprits that prevent you from ever losing weight or body fat. In chapter 11, you'll uncover the champion toxin, which may surprise you. Chapter 12 describes the three toxins we commonly consume that our bodies do not recognize as food. In chapter 13, you'll learn the differences between three stimulants that disrupt homeostasis.

Part Four: Dr. Healthnut Real

Part Four helps you shift from fake to real foods. Chapter 14 demystifies the three healthy food principles. You'll also learn about the three real food types. Chapter 15 teaches you how to eat like a healthnut. You'll know which foods are better for you. In chapter 16, you'll learn how to self-test to assess which foods work well by listening to your body.

Part 5: Dr. Healthnut Action

Part Five instructs you to take action—the healthnut way! You'll create your roadmap for the lifestyle that works for you. Chapter 17 shows you the

Healthnut Life by providing the healthy lifestyle principles that you adopt into your personalized program. In chapter 18, you'll create your own plan based on the principles you align with from the book. You (not me, not anyone else!) decide what you will eat or won't eat. The program will provide the framework to encompass whichever foods you specifically include over the seasons of your life, and as long as you are choosing to incorporate real food into your lifestyle plan, you will inevitably and even immediately see healthier results. Finally, chapter 19 summarizes the ultimate perspective for sharing your newfound lifestyle.

Look, I know what it's like to struggle with lifestyle and health issues. I've wrestled with chronic pain and disease on one extreme and have experienced healing and vitality on the other. The choices we make on a daily basis add up over time. When you make healthier choices, it's like you are providing your body the chance to be optimized, healed, and restored.

YOUR WHOLENESS

Ultimately, my goal is to provide the best of my advice and experience for you. To accomplish this massive task, I rely on my faith in God to really help me. My prayer is that you would not only identify some great tips, but ultimately experience the wholeness that God has designed for you. Wholeness is a complex topic and incorporates multiple dimensions of health—spirit, soul, and body. Don't worry if you're not ready to broach this complex subject in one day—or one week, or one month. I believe that by just taking one step, and then another, to eat healthier, you'll *get well, restore hope,* and *be alive!*

What are you waiting for? Join me in the epic shift to *healthnut-ize* the world.

PART ONE:

DR. HEALTHNUT WORLD

HEALTHNUT CHOICE

Have you ever wondered why obesity and being overweight, collectively known as "OB," continues to be an epidemic in our nation and throughout the world despite each year's influx of new diets? According to the US Department of Health and Human Services, more than two in three adults are overweight or obese—and more than one in three adults are considered to be obese.[4] One in three US kids aged 2–19 struggle with OB, which is triple the figure thirty years ago. They are also twice as likely to die by age 55 compared to children with a healthy weight. According to the American Public Health Association, the direct costs of medical care and indirect costs of lost productivity, etc., totals hundreds of billions of dollars annually.[5] Furthermore, the Mayo Clinic estimates that nearly 7 out of 10 Americans are on prescription drugs.[6] Integrative and lifestyle physicians are bombarded with the rampant growth of lifestyle diseases stemming from OB.

RAMPANT OB

Dr. Bill Wilson, an integrative medical specialist who addresses weight and body composition issues, has conducted body composition measurements on over 18,000 patients. Dr. Wilson points out that *overweight* is defined as "excess body weight" and *obesity* as "excess body fat."[7] For those struggling with OB, excess body weight or excess body fat is identical in terms of health consequences. A tremendous healthcare tragedy arising from OB has been brewing globally for decades, and the associated problems and solutions are more complex than ever.

For example, some patients' disease is masked by the guise of being outwardly "thin" but inwardly "fat." So is the internally OB person better off than the outwardly OB person? To add to the perplexity, a recent study in the *Journal of the American Medical Association* (*JAMA*) claims that those slightly overweight with a higher Body Mass Index (BMI) than non-overweight individuals have a lower death rate.[8] However, the results of this study fail to consider other ramifications. For example, what is the benefit of having a lower death rate if you live a lower quality of life with OB and have to take a prescription drug? Or, how many of the participants in this study were already on prescription drugs? Compare these results to the reality of those who might live one year less but die without a debilitating or chronic disease. You may realize that you care about what maximizes and prolongs the *quality* of life, not the *quantity* of years lived! You want to feel and live *better* and not just *longer*.

Certainly, the OB dilemma contributes to preventable deaths associated with cardiovascular disease, cancer, diabetes, and other chronic conditions. Do you think there is a correlation between the 69.2% of the population struggling with these mostly lifestyle-related diseases and the almost 70% of the population on prescription drugs?

And what about the other one-third of the population—you know, the healthnuts?[9] Why don't they struggle with OB? Well, healthnuts endeavor to reduce their exposure to the negative effects of toxicity to virtually eliminate the chances of OB and many related lifestyle diseases. This does not mean healthnuts are perfect and experience vitality in every area of life during every second of the day. There are other factors involved in health that go beyond the food aspect. However, it's undeniable that what we put in our mouths is a significant contributor to our health and vitality. Wanting to be a healthnut is really about the *desire* to live a higher quality life and to learn how to live it consistently—for years to come.

HEALTHNUTS...

- Avoid lifestyle practices that lead to OB.
- Experience a lifelong freedom from OB.
- Are not really crazy...they just want to be healthy!

THREE MAJOR CAUSES OF OB

CAUSE #1: BODY TOXICITY

There are three major causes of OB: body toxicity, soul toxicity, and info toxicity. The first major cause of OB is body toxicity. How do you know if you have body toxicity? You can take a quick test to determine whether or not you have body toxicity. Check any of the following symptoms below that you experience regularly.

BODY TOXICITY SYMPTOMS

- ❏ bad breath
- ❏ brain fog
- ❏ dry skin
- ❏ body odor
- ❏ pain
- ❏ dandruff
- ❏ fatigue
- ❏ joint pain
- ❏ belly fat
- ❏ acne
- ❏ sleep problems
- ❏ constipation
- ❏ digestive difficulties
- ❏ bloating/gas
- ❏ food addiction

Now, I don't mean to scare you or point the finger at you. Whether or not you checked any or all of the above, the chances are that you will experience toxicity at some point in your life. It's not the temporal body toxicity symptoms listed above that are of concern, but the pervasive, slow-growing pattern of systemic toxicity over time that is most damaging. Let's take a look at some of the factors that cause body toxicity.

BODY TOXICITY SOURCE #1: UNCONTROLLABLE FACTORS

An uncontrollable factor is a factor that exposes your body to toxicity against your will. An example of an uncontrollable factor is when you inhale or ingest environmental pollution while traveling or even crossing the street. Another example is breathing secondhand smoke in a public air space. A third (less significant) example is your genetics and the (more significant) modified impact on your genetics from your lifestyle choices and your environment. Each of these uncontrollable factors may influence your level of body toxicity at any given phase of your life.

It is said that what you inherit will not change. How much of a role does genetics have in influencing the expression of your personal body toxicity? Your genetics account for about between 20%–30% of your health (some researchers place that figure as low as 5%). The other 70%–80% of your health outcomes are related to your lifestyle choices. There are now many uncontrollable factors that may impact your level of body toxicity. Yes, your DNA can be switched on to express disease characteristics, sometimes without your control.

The field that studies these genetic factors is called "epigenetics." Epigenetics is more than just understanding your genetics. Epigenetics also explores the genetic expression and dynamic response of your body to diet, lifestyle, behavior, and toxins through chemical alterations.[10] Your genetic expression is a critical lifestyle element because it tells your body how to function in our environment. If your genes intend to transform to a monstrosity via uncontrollable factors, you may experience more dysfunction in your body, one of which is OB. In the medical community, patients who have unknowingly been exposed to abnormally high levels of lead and mercury experience the uncontrollable factor of toxic element exposure. Additionally, evidence emerges that chemicals such as pesticides and BPA are linked to metabolic dysfunction, insulin resistance, and ultimately predict OB.[11] The overabundance of exposure to these toxins may increase the risk factor of complex diseases.

HEALTHNUTS...

- Recognize the importance of uncontrollable factors in body toxicity.
- Understand genetics has less influence on OB than lifestyle practices.
- Respect the larger role of the epigenetic risk for OB.

BODY TOXICITY SOURCE #2: CONTROLLABLE FACTORS

A controllable factor is a factor that's within your power; you can choose whether you allow that source of toxicity into your body. For example, one controllable factor is deciding what to eat—for example, whether you choose to snack on potato chips or on peanut butter and celery. A second controllable factor is what you put on your skin—for example, whether you regularly use spray-on tans or vitamin E. A third controllable factor is what products you bring into your household—for example, whether your laundry consistently comes in contact with chemically enhanced dryer sheets or all-natural detergent. Keep in mind that although there are varying levels of healthy and unhealthy, what's most important is taking steps in the right direction to create a higher quality of life.

In the US, similar to other developed nations, the leading source of OB is malnutrition. How is this possible in a land with such easy access to food? Because we have increased the amount of food but decreased the nutritional quality. We spend more on food that is lacking key nutrients, which causes an overfed form of malnourishment. During a recent conversation with my friend Dr. Jacob Tietelbaum, who is an integrative physician expert in lifestyle medicine, he disclosed the truth of nutrition in one simple phrase: "Malnutrition is at an all-time high."[12] Surprisingly, although we have more food availability throughout the world today than probably ever before in history, our cells are still starving for fuel.

If you want quality food, you will either have to pay for it or farm it yourself. Thankfully, there are agricultural movements aimed at making farming more sustainable and ecological through efficient food-growing systems such as hydroponics or fish repopulation strategies. Ultimately, there is no way around accessing high quality food sources. More than ever, you must make a choice to be conscious about the foods you purchase as a small part of creating a market demand for healthier food. Otherwise, you may continue to struggle for the rest of your life, both personally, because of your own weight and health issues, and more generally, with not being able to find healthy food. The choice is yours.

WHERE TO BEGIN?

Choosing the wrong food leads to an increase in weight and Body Mass Index (BMI). BMI is often the standard used to determine a healthy height and weight balance ratio. However, BMI is one of the worst indicators of overall health. Regardless of your level of systemic body toxicity, one of the most accurate methods to measure your body composition is through a Dual-energy X-ray absorptiometry (DEXA) scan. A DEXA scan accurately snaps a big picture of your body composition by measuring bone mineral density. You might say, "Wait a minute I don't want a dose of radiation." I don't either, but rest assured that a DEXA scan actually uses less radiation than a typical chest x-ray.[13]

A less invasive and an inexpensive option for determining your lean and fat mass ratio is body fat calipers. When I was a professional fitness trainer many years ago, I always began with a new client by taking their baseline body fat and lean mass measurements. The clients' goal was to reduce negative body fat levels, and thereby decrease inches in pant, dress, and waist sizes. Measuring your body fat levels is far superior to weight measurements alone. It's possible to lose weight, but increase unhealthy fat mass, which will not help your goal to be healthy.

Also, keep in mind that losing weight and becoming thin does not always equate to health and vitality. You can be thin but have toxic fat buildup around your organs. What you want is a balance of a healthy weight and body fat ratio that works for your height, frame, and makeup—the ideal you! The real you is not about comparing yourself to anyone. It's about maximizing your God-given health to optimal function. Crash dieting, or bouncing from diet to diet, is about the worst thing you can do to be healthy and lose either weight or fat.

HEALTHNUTS...

- Acknowledge the importance of controllable factors.
- Avoid foods that cause malnourishment.
- Focus on balancing body composition and reducing inches instead of weight.

CAUSE #2: SOUL TOXICITY

The second major cause of OB is soul toxicity. I define the soul as your mind, will, and emotions. There are soulish aspects of OB that include your mind and emotions; science is only now beginning to address the influence of the mind and emotional aspects of the soul on the physical body. A recent analysis of obesity-related behaviors in 67 peer-reviewed articles from 1976 to 2013 found that neurocognitive dysfunction creates reductions in activity, poor eating habits, and higher intakes of food.[14] It is plausible that the combination of OB and neurocognitive decline energizes the vicious cycle of a negative soul feedback loop. In other words, effects from a negative soul contribute repeatedly to poor choices with bad physical outcomes. Most of this research is tangible but there are other soul-related factors that are less physically apparent.

THE PLACEBO REALITY

Ted Kapchuk, Associate Professor of Medicine at Harvard, believes that what has been called the placebo effect, or the success of a harmless but ineffectual treatment simply because the patient cognitively believes that it is working, may be authentic—a belief that parallels what some of the top scientists may also sheepishly and quietly admit. Kapchuk acknowledges the limitations in research and does not necessarily claim to exactly know how the placebo works.[15] If the placebo effect, however, is real, what is most important to take away is that the mind (or intellect), will, and emotion of an individual is an influential part of health, even if we don't yet fully understand how.

During one of my international trips, I explored this topic with Dr. Frans Cronje, who is a world-renowned lecturer on the interdisciplinary nature of medical science and healing. In a conversation over breakfast, Dr. Cronje wondered aloud why unexplainable things could happen in medicine. During one intense moment in our interaction, he exclaimed in his stern but articulate, convincing tone, "It's because the placebo is real!"[16] Up until that point, I've always thought placebo was anecdotal. It was not science. It was the unexplained that just happened by chance. It was the sugar pill phenomenon.

He then dropped a rather large term: psychoneuroimmunoendocrinology. "What is that?" I inquired. Essentially, he explained, psychoneuroimmunoendocrinology (PNIE, for short) is an entire field that attempts to explain the interrelations between the mind and body. It claims that your mind and body communicate, and in that communication, they may influence one another.[17] This is the very reason Dr. Cronje postulates that a branded placebo sugar pill and branded drug achieves better success than a non-branded placebo or a non-branded drug. The mind-body gap in our understanding is closed by the fact that the placebo is acting as an authentic representation of the unconscious conditioning of belief along with a conscious expectation of benefit in an individual's mind.[18] Their research contributes understanding to what I call the placebo reality. Expect to see more research on the placebo reality in the coming years.

MIND-BODY CONNECTION

You may already be familiar with mind-body medicine, which emerged in the latter half of the twentieth century and is related to the placebo reality. Far more significant than mind-body medicine alone, I believe the next big wave that twenty-first century science will explore is spirituality. Some believe, including myself, that there is a spiritual dimension, separate from the soul and body, which interacts and communicates with the soul and body. Dr. Harold Koenig, who is the co-director of Duke's Center for Spirituality, Theology, and Health, describes the importance of addressing spiritual issues in healthcare as more studies continue to identify the relationship between spirituality and better health.[19] However, spirituality is more challenging to understand, observe, and measure from a scientific perspective, at least in terms of the frameworks we are familiar with in science or even in anecdotal evidence today.

(Because of that complexity, I do not include much spirituality in this book. Spirituality and health needs its own book, even multiple books, to begin to ask the right questions in the process of understanding its health-related dynamics. However, I've attempted to address it in *Leading Wholeness*, a multidimensional theoretical framework for leaders and health professionals to positively impact the health of nations with spirit, soul, and body.)

So how does the placebo reality affect your mind and body? Consider that some pharmaceutical drugs may only need to achieve a minimum of 1% effectiveness above placebo to be approved in clinical trials. Did you know the placebo effect might be as high as 30% or more? Wellness coaching is a health framework to exercise and work with your mind to proactively and positively influence your physical body by focusing on lifestyle solutions that are meaningful, motivating, and manageable.

This is nothing new in terms of health communication. World-renowned psychiatrist, Dr. Daniel Amen, in his book *Change Your Brain, Change Your Body*, describes the benefits of the brain's influence on the body. I've learned from Dr. Amen that when the mind harmonizes with the body, patients get the best results.[20] It's no different for you. Your mind is the most powerful influencer of your body.

HEALTHNUTS...

- Know there is a possibility of experiencing the placebo reality.
- Acknowledge the impact PNIE has on brain, hormone, and body weight.
- Understand that a positive mind-set may improve success for a healthy body.

EMOTION-BODY CONNECTION

The other half of the soul connection to your body is your emotional outlet. Science is obliging, as researchers continue to explore the connection between biological actions such as food consumption and the emotional aspects of the mind.[21] In my work coaching physicians and organizations to help their patients achieve a healthy lifestyle and weight, I've found emotions are influential on both spectrums, whether positively or negatively. Depression, anxiety, fear, worry, anger, and frustration will prevent success in overcoming OB.

Ultimately, negative emotions may drive us to seek new health professionals, new diets, or even harmful substances to remedy our health challenges. A major problem with today's diet industry is that it does not take into account your long-term success—even though long-term success is one of the biggest obstacles in dieting! Your emotions play a powerful role in accepting or rejecting this lifetime plan, whether positive or negative.

There are entire fields of study dedicated to comprehending the connection between emotional status and OB. One of my favorite books that I encountered in graduate studies was *Emotional Intelligence* by *New York Times* best-selling author Daniel Goleman. Dr. Goleman was the first to emphasize that healthy emotional expression must be considered as important as sheer IQ alone.[22] Your Emotional Quotient (EQ) is a measure of your emotional abilities. Emotional Intelligence (EI) is a complementary measure of emotional insight and understanding. A good percentage of your EQ and EI self-leadership capacity is related to the influence of your surrounding environment.[23] For example, if you put a child in a negative learning environment, their chance of success is much lower than a child who was placed in an area of positive emotional support.

Dr. Ben Carson is a famous neurosurgeon responsible for the first separation of twins conjoined at the head. As a young boy, Dr. Carson did not have a present father. However, he had a strong mother and supportive teachers. Although he was not in the best possible atmosphere, there was a positive system and strong accountability when he was growing up.[24] It could be argued that he had a gift that helped him supersede the negative constructs of his environment. That gift would not have fully developed had he not had the right support, encouragement, and accountability. This is why a supportive community is vital to health success.

Your emotions are real. Don't allow anyone to downplay your positive emotions. Sometimes, there will be an unknown, a question mark, or an unidentified factor that will bring you success in finding your health goals. You may not always be able to put a finger on what caused a considerable shift in your life—it may have been something you read, one word from a close friend or colleague, or even one small, successful eating achievement that lasts for years—but one thing is all it takes to never give up. It might take some time, but with God's help and your willingness to keep moving forward, positive emotional support will be a strength for you.

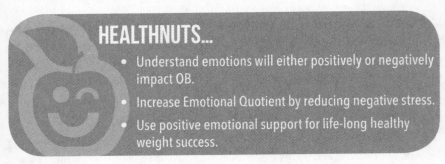

HEALTHNUTS...

- Understand emotions will either positively or negatively impact OB.
- Increase Emotional Quotient by reducing negative stress.
- Use positive emotional support for life-long healthy weight success.

CAUSE #3: INFO TOXICITY

DIET CONFUSION?

Did you know that the diet industry profits off your struggle with OB—through something I call info toxicity? Info toxicity is the overabundance of conflicting information that causes confusion from the influx of new diets annually. Consumers spend $61 billion per year in the US alone, just on diets.[25] The diet industry develops a new diet fad, celebrity solution, fantastic food, or beverage product daily. Keeping the market full of so-called new and improved solutions is how they increase revenues every year. The diet industry is incredibly savvy and knows exactly which buttons to push to get you into their program. They know 99% of people will fail long term on their diet programs, and will require a new program to keep them motivated.

But the money-driven industry will never be able to offer you a long-term solution because you weren't designed to fit someone else's program. You need a plan that was designed for you—a plan that is unlike anyone else's.

STRUGGLING WITH OB

If you battle with OB, is it your fault entirely? No! Part of your situation is your choice, and the other part is a lack of quality information. The knowledge and information to live healthy is either kept from you or you have not discovered it yet. You may know what you need to do, but if you don't have the resources to do it, you'll never be successful. The majority of the burden of making food more accessible and affordable rests on the producers or gatekeepers to our health, which include the agricultural industry, food production, manufacturing of products and services, media and advertising, and food delivery systems.

We can change this current system with a grassroots approach by linking our arms together in cohesive unity to demand the healthiest and most eco-friendly choices to be readily available to each of us, everywhere. Essentially, we all become healthnuts of some sort, with different levels and approaches.

If you want to be a healthnut, you deserve a fair shot to be healthy for life. Remember, being a healthnut is not about being crazy, or excessive, but simply maximizing the quality of your life by making healthier choices daily. It's not just for the elite, it's for those of you who want to be healthy, for your families, and for your coworkers. You have a right to be healthy! You have a right to good food! You have a right to know that what you eat will either harm or help your body! At the very least, you should have a right to choose to eat healthily or not!

You may think you can just go on the Internet and research your answers, but there is simply too much misinformation and over-information to be able to navigate a plan that is right for you. How do you know that information you've read is accurate? How do you know it will work for you? What is the source? For every study that shows the benefits of x, y, or z, there is more than likely another study that shows everything but the benefits of x, y, and z!

We're living in a culture, even in the scientific community, that prizes knowledge. To live healthily, however, we need more than knowledge. We must move from knowledge to insight to wisdom on the right path at the right time with the right support community. A colleague and mentor to me, Dr. Titus Parker, who is a brilliant anti-aging physician, frequently states during his lectures, "Real information costs something."[26] The investments you make in educating yourself with real information are priceless.

HEALTHNUTS...

- Are not duped by the diet industry.
- Participate in lobbying for true information about healthy food accessibility.
- Seek authentic health information from knowledgeable experts and use it.

HEALTHNUT SIMPLICITY

New diet books come and go. Most of the diets in the marketplace are tested on a select population group, and there are always tremendous successes and notable failures. It's just like infomercials promising the greatest new gadget; they always have the disclaimer that these are exceptional results and not the norm. That's because the diets do work—but only for the people that stick to them!

DIET CYCLES

Too many diets, however, are far too difficult to "stick to," or maintain over the long-term. This is especially true when there is deprivation of any form, as the Oregon Research Institute found in a study of food deprivation and weight loss.[27] People who were deprived of food for a period of time usually go back to the food they consumed prior to their diet—maybe that explains why people tend to gain weight back after dieting. Similarly, a large percentage of contestants on popular weight-loss shows gain weight back after going through the program.

Healthnuts understand the secret to lifestyle success is in their daily decisions that add, rather than detract, from their health. Comparatively, somebody unconcerned about their health may say, "Well, I've smoked for years, and I don't have any health problems." But how does that person know whether their body responds positively to an unnatural chemical? Do you want to gamble penny wise but pound foolish with your health?

It's true that there may be some things you can do that are unhealthy and yet you won't immediately see any negative results—at least, any results that you can see or feel on a surface level without in-depth scrutiny. But how do you really know that a bad habit does not have unforeseen consequences over time? Doctors don't know everything; a clean bill of health from your physician doesn't necessarily mean that everything is okay. There are thousands of lab tests you can take, but that doesn't mean these tests are always accurate. Your physician-ordered lab tests may come out great even though you still struggle with OB or another disease.

It certainly doesn't help that doctors are ceaselessly inundated with the latest pharmaceutical literature and promotion bonuses. Drug companies spend millions on lobbying and incentivizing physicians to tout their latest weight-loss drug.[28] And that's just one type of drug! During my on-site nutritional consults with physicians, I would often see the "pharma reps" competing with me for my time. It's a money game, and there is certainly hot competition for the trillion—yes, *trillion*—dollar healthcare market.

Some physicians are eager to quickly write a prescription and send a patient on their way with a brief, "Oh, just take this pill, and you'll be fine." They don't attempt to get to the root reality. Often, they are being forced by the current healthcare systems to reach a high quota of patients per hour and are thus constantly pressed for time. The exact situation is heavily dependent on specialty, training, practice group, and other factors. Now, please note that there are absolutely many healthcare providers who genuinely care and have done an outstanding job even in the most dire circumstance when acute interventions like surgery or drugs are necessary. My point instead is that physicians should not necessarily be the first line of defense for lifestyle-related healthcare issues, since many must work within the status quo. However, as a healthpreneur, my job is to challenge the status quo! I want the best for you—not the status quo!

Regardless of what anyone says, your cause for illness will be unique; your challenge is to discover why you may struggle with OB or other health issues. Diet promoters know that, as long as you don't find your own unique cause for illness, you will be back for more of their products. They think you don't have the fortitude to live a continual, healthy lifestyle; they might even think you are ignorant, based on their past monetary successes. I believe something different. You may have failed with other diets, but you are ready to overcome, no matter what it takes. You want to see your children and even your children's children. You want to be vibrant and healthy.

The good news is that your body was made to repair itself. When you cut yourself, what happens if you provide the proper care? It heals. Did you do the healing? No, you removed the interference and supported your body's innate healing mechanisms to maximize the recovery process. So let's remove some more interference!

HEALTHNUTS...

- Know the secret to healthy weight is found in daily habits and choices.
- Take initiative to learn about individualized health.
- Don't do the diet cycle but the lifestyle cycle—forever.

DIET MARKETING TECHNIQUES

What are the hidden marketing techniques of the weight management industry?

Perhaps the most common hidden marketing technique in the diet industry promises that you will lose weight. But the body weight statistic does not tell the whole story. The marketing might promise that you'll lose 30 pounds in 30 days or 7 pounds in 7 days. These messages fulfill our nation's immediate-gratification syndrome that always wants fast results! But what are the health ramifications from such drastic weight loss? What other associated health problems are caused? What are the long-term implications? If you lose the weight that quickly, you will almost inevitably gain it back, slow but sure. Each time you diet cycle, both your metabolism and your ability to burn energy and store fat is disrupted. One interesting study from the *The New England Journal of Medicine* has demonstrated that hormone and appetite disruption occurs with weight loss.[29] That probably doesn't bother the marketers of the diet industry, however, because they know that the more weight people gain back, the more likely they will come back for another diet.

If you want to break free of the unhealthy rhythm, like healthnuts do, you will have to make a lifetime lifestyle decision. You will have think, *What changes am I willing to make, not just for thirty days, but for life?* You will have to change your daily routine. You will have to make some different choices in how and what you eat. It's always going to be more difficult at the beginning, but if you are willing to begin the journey of new choices, you will have long-term success.

LET'S SIMPLIFY THE DIET COMPLEXITY

Diet philosophies change constantly, because there is no one-size-fits-all plan. Rather, every individual is unique. The secret is finding out what works for you in every given season of your life. You can take two people with the same height, weight, gender, metabolism, and even blood chemistry, put them side-by-side, and they may still require two completely different solutions to OB. We know this from studies done on twins with very similar genetic characteristics whose individual lifestyle choices created quite different health outcomes. That's because the cause of OB is different for each person—and so the remedy will be unique, too! You have to find the solution that's going to work for your individual biochemistry, biology, biomechanics, biodiversity, psychology, and neurological, immune, digestive, metabolic, and hormonal systems. I bet that sounds really complicated to you. That's why the Healthnut Life is all about answering this question: How can we simplify this diet complexity and focus on behaviors we enjoy to naturally yield healthy outcomes?

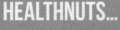

HEALTHNUTS...

- Avoid drastic weight-loss habits which produce unhealthy long-term consequences.
- Recognize their individuality and use it to their advantage toward a healthier lifestyle.
- Are answering this question: How do we simplify the diet complexity?

THE HEALTHNUT LIFE

Healthnuts naturally live a lifestyle that is conducive to maintaining a healthy weight. How do they do it? The answer is in what I call the "Healthnut Life." In reality, the Healthnut Life is not a diet—it's a lifestyle. *Diet* often implies short-term weight loss but long-term uncertainty. *Diet* also sounds like "death and that's it"—die-it. I don't know about you, but I'd rather focus on life! Healthnuts pick healthy eating principles that work for them for life. Yes, some of those principles are found in certain diets—such as caloric restriction, eliminating gluten or dairy, and exercise. But the difference is that instead of being fixated on one principle for a short amount of time, healthnuts use all types of lifestyle activities to accomplish their goals of lifelong health maintenance. That's the beauty of the Healthnut Life, you have lots of options and you can find one that works best for you.

COACHING MIND-SET

The formula for lifelong healthy weight incorporates coaching methodology, motivational interviewing, and the practical action steps that you choose. Researchers continue to explore the power of coaching and motivational interviewing through studies in healthcare settings to determine whether they support participation, empathy, and personal goal-setting for overcoming lifestyle challenges.[30] You see, when you are in charge of your lifestyle choices, you will commit for life versus being told for five weeks what to eat and how to walk and then going back to old habits when the five weeks are up. I'm going to share lots of tips and techniques that healthnuts use, but, as I said at the beginning, it's up to you to choose which ones you incorporate into your routine.

HEALTHNUT LIFE STEPS

STEP #1: RATE YOUR HEALTHNUT INSPIRATION

For you to accomplish any goal in life, you must first assess if you are truly motivated or inspired to make that change. I've discovered that self-awareness at any given stage in life is a master key to accomplishing anything worthwhile. I've developed a simple self-analysis test[31] that I call your Healthnut Inspire. You can rate your appropriate level for any health or life desire with the following chart. Here's an example:

| Reflection | Consideration | Anticipation | Engagement | Preservation |
| 1 | 2 | 3 | 4 | 5 |

1. Reflection: I am reflecting on changing my _____ but not ready.

2. Consideration: I am considering changing my _____ in the future.

3. Anticipation: I am anticipating I will make _____ changes soon.

4. Engagement: I am actively engaged in *diet lifestyle* changes now.

5. Preservation: I am preserving my _____ changes for life.

My number is ____4____.

Let's try a little exercise and see where you are at this moment. Rate yourself in terms of your desire for eating healthy and being at a healthy weight on a scale of 1 to 5, based on which space you fill in.

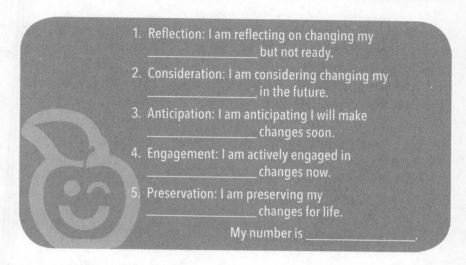

1. Reflection: I am reflecting on changing my
   _____ but not ready.
2. Consideration: I am considering changing my
   _____ in the future.
3. Anticipation: I am anticipating I will make
   _____ changes soon.
4. Engagement: I am actively engaged in
   _____ changes now.
5. Preservation: I am preserving my
   _____ changes for life.
   My number is _____.

STEP #2: IDENTIFY YOUR HEALTHNUT *AHA!*

I've invested thousands of hours coaching health professionals, business-es, and clients and I guarantee your success depends on identifying your *Aha!* moment. The *Aha!* I am referring to is like an expression of triumph and de-lighted discovery—you've identified what works for you—and it's a glimpse of bliss and serendipity.

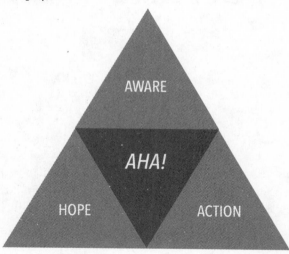

Your Healthnut *Aha!* stands for your ideal awareness state, desired hope, and practical action steps. You need to have an awareness of who you are and who you want to be. You need to have hope to create specific goals that help you get to your ideal vision. You need to have an action plan to reach that hope. Yes, this approach has to do with your mind-set. We'll cover this in more detail later on, but for right now, you can remember how to create your Healthnut *Aha!* by using the formula below:

1. A = Aware: identifying *what you actually want*, your dream, your overall ideal vision for your health.

2. H = Hope: your specific goal to be accomplished within a specific time frame.

3. A = Action: the practical steps you'll take to reach your hope goals.

STEP #3: CHOOSE YOUR HEALTHNUT FANS

To accomplish your *Aha!* most successfully, you'll need to have support; I call this support your "Healthnut Fans." You need three main fans:

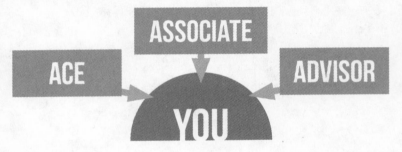

1. Ace: The ace is your expert.

2. Associate: The associate is your participating partner.

3. Advisor: The advisor is your mentor.

Fans are vital because they provide support for your journey, encouragement for your successes, and accountability for your challenges. Again, we'll have more to say about your Healthnut Fans in the final section.

REAL LIFE

What is the best diet or lifestyle? The best diet for you is one that maximizes your metabolism, reduces the effects of aging, rejuvenates your soul, inspires your spirit, produces preventive health characteristics in your body, balances your hormones and digestive system, and enhances your overall well-being. What is that diet? That is the million-dollar healthnut question.

This is what you, and you alone, will discover.

That is why you must invest in discovering your health individuality. If you delay this process, you delay realizing your unique wellness map. The Healthnut Life provides you the blueprint to discover and implement your lifelong lifestyle plan for a healthy weight. So, if you haven't taken the leap to become a healthnut, time is not on your side! Do it now!

HEALTHNUTS...

- Find the lifestyle plan targeted to interests, preferences, and lifestyle.
- Adjust the lifestyle plan with each phase of life to maintain a healthy weight.
- Don't view eating healthy as dieting but as part of a new lifestyle.

STRUGGLING WITH HEALTH ISSUES, COSTLY MEDICAL BILLS, OR WEIGHT GAIN ANXIETY?
JOIN THE HEALTHNUT COMMUNITY BY VISITING **DRHEALTHNUT.COM**
TO HELP YOU GET BACK ON THE PATH TO HEALTH, HEALING, AND WHOLENESS NOW!

SCAN TO VISIT DRHEALTHNUT.COM

PART TWO:

DR. HEALTHNUT DECODE

4

HEALTHNUT MAJORS

Before we jump into this chapter, I want to provide a few quick definitions and basic explanations that will be vital to your understanding as we diagnose specific diets. If you know them already—wonderful! If you don't, here's the breakdown.

MAJOR VERSUS MINOR

There are two types of nutrients that we need to eat in order to survive: macronutrients and micronutrients. As their names indicate, we need macronutrients in much larger amounts than we need micronutrients. Macronutrients, then, comprise the bulk of the food that we eat. The three main macronutrients are carbohydrates, proteins, and fats (see the three major diets later in the chapter!).

Carbohydrates are the main energy providers for our body and are mostly composed of sugar, fiber, and starches. If carbohydrates aren't burned as energy, they may be converted from glucose and stored as fat in our body. Although basically all foods contain carbohydrates to some extent, the foods with the highest amount of carbs include healthier fruits and vegetables, any unhealthy sugary products, cereals, crackers, cakes, flours, bread products, and potato products.

Proteins are formed by a multitude of amino acids, the body's building blocks. Our organs, muscles, skin, hair, and even nails are built from and repaired by proteins. Proteins transport, message, structure, and protect the body and are fueled in their work by carbohydrates and fats. Foods with a high amount of protein include meat, dairy products, fish products, beans, eggs, and nuts and seeds.

Fat is a critical macronutrient for metabolic structure and function and acts as an ideal source of energy. During lean times, the body pulls on its fat reserves for energy, converting it into glucose. There are two main types of fat, saturated and unsaturated. Foods that are high in saturated fats may come from both animal and plant sources and are solid at room temperature, including meat products, dairy products, egg products, and vegetarian-based coconut oil. Foods that are high in unsaturated fats come from vegetable sources and include less-desirable omega-6 fatty acids from vegetable oils like peanut or corn oil and more-desirable omega-3 fatty acids from oily fish like sockeye salmon.

Most people, however, are doing just fine on the amount of their macronutrients (although balance can be another issue!). It's the micronutrients where consumption tends to decline. Micronutrients are small dietary compounds, chiefly vitamins, minerals, fatty acid compounds like antioxidants and phytochemicals, which are not produced by the body and yet perform vital functions. Most of us know about the benefits of micronutrients like vitamin A or iron, but lesser-known micronutrients are no less important. Take polyphenols for an example, which are powerful molecules found in higher concentrations in spices, fruits, nuts, vegetables, and seeds. Polyphenols are very complex and are indicated to reduce inflammation, improve brain health, slow oxidative and free radical damage in aging, and reduce the risk factors for many lifestyle related diseases. The major categories include phenolic acids, lignins, stillbenes, and the popular flavonoids.[32]

THE TRUTH ABOUT DIETS

I recently had the pleasure of sitting down with the executive of one of the top international media companies to discuss a few projects. John (not his actual name) has a bio that reads like a *Who's Who* of the famous. From leadership gurus to iconic pastors, from entertainment executives to just about every top-of-mind celebrity I could think of, John has provided his valuable input and insight for their projects. With all of his success, what impressed me most about him (besides his humility) was his familiarity with top diets. We briefly discussed the major confusion that accompanies the release of a new diet book. Each new diet seems to add to the confusion. One of the reasons he confided in me is because his wife struggled with her diet over the years. Could her challenge be that very few experts voice the truth about dieting?

That is, the truth that there is really no one diet that works for everyone! Each of us must uncover our unique personalized diet or lifestyle plan.

That sounds simple enough. Why is it so challenging?

It's so challenging because even once you discover the diet that works best for you, it's difficult to implement that diet regularly in your life. Although some diets may work well, others are moderately successful at best, and dangerous at worst. In my consulting work with health professionals, I've observed a wide variety of diets that are recommended for their patients. The sheer variety of options can be quite overwhelming.

Recently, I posted an article on a business forum I participate in to receive some feedback on dieting. The article promoted a specific type of diet, mainly a higher carbohydrate focus with a lower amount of protein and fat. I asked the group what they thought of the diet. I received answers all over the board from health experts. If even these health professionals are divided on which diets are healthy, it's no wonder that most people, without the benefit of a degree in health or nutrition, are confused about what's the best diet!

After reviewing many diet themes spanning both diet eras and geographic regions, I've discovered consistent patterns for healthy eating, activity, and weight monitoring. Although I've tried to specifically address many of the diet themes for you, most diets can be generally categorized as a modified caloric restriction, a fasting, an energy-boosting, or a food-elimination process, according to long-term diet analysis.

Unfortunately, the statistics report that only 2% of dieters maintain the new weight or lifestyle for life.[33] Don't be a part of the 98% that cannot maintain their weight or even 2% that go on diets and succeed! Do away with the statistics altogether! You are not a statistic. You are a champion, and with the appropriate food remedy you will discover and maintain a healthy weight for life.

HEALTHNUTS...

- Avoid extreme diets and opt for saying yes to a personalized lifestyle plan.
- Lead health transformation rather than follow crash diet fads.
- Discover a unique health remedy that works forever.

I've summarized below what I believe are the 10 major diet themes that people attempt.

SAD Diet	3 Major Diets	3 Popular Diets	3 Specialty Diets
Healthnuts avoid the Standard American Diet (SAD Diet)	1. Carb-focused 2. Protein-focused 3. Fat-focused	1. Vegetarian 2. Fasting 3. Metabolic	1. High-plant 2. Gluten-free 3. Athletic

Let's look at these in more detail.

SAD DIET

PROCESSED AND FAST FOODS

The Standard American Diet (SAD) is really just that—sad. This diet includes fast food, snacks, unhealthy drinks, and quick, easy, and convenient unhealthy foods. Our culture encourages this eating pattern. Turn on the TV and you'll see commercials that promote eating foods that cost peanuts to produce but are sold for a fortune. If you really understand how inexpensive it is to produce this garbage, you would be astonished that people consume it at high rates and high prices. It's also a form of population control in my opinion. If they, whoever "they" is, can keep you sick, keep you struggling from OB, keep you from knowing the truth about what's going to keep you well, you'll be the fodder for their money-grubbing production. You can change that pattern today with a renewed focus to eliminate SAD.

Don't feel bad if you are caught in the web of sick food. I consumed mostly SAD when I was younger. During my early years, my mom forced me to eat a moderately healthy diet. But as a college student, freed from the shackles of home life, I frequented fast-food joints. One summer, I ate two double whoppers with cheese, lettuce, mayonnaise, and fries for lunch every single day! The really sad part is my external physique did not show it. That's because the fake food is slow poison and may not demonstrate the immediate health consequences. Yes, I may have been ripped (about 5–7% body fat), but my organs were screaming, "We are unhealthy!" Although I haven't struggled with

OB personally, it's reported in the *British Medical Journal* that those who have predisposition toward excess fat deposits will react epigenetically to the over-consumption of unhealthy SAD foods.[34]

Today, you couldn't pay me to eat that sewage. In fact, I cringe when I hear one of my family members say they want to grab-and-go with some fast food. "What! You're not going to eat that trash, are you?" I exclaim. Yes, my response may be a little harsh, but at least I am honest and care about their—and your—wellbeing. Hey, that's the coach in me!

SAD REALITY

Is the rise in hypnotic, stomach-satisfying fake food all our fault? *The Journal of the American Medical Association* reports in one analysis that fast food consumption increases with fast-food availability.[35] In other words, if you live near processed and fast-food restaurants, you are more likely to consume their seductions. That seems pretty logical, right? On the flip side of the coin, if there are not healthier food choices available, which has occasionally been the case in my life, then it's incredibly easy to succumb to those tempting de-sires. That's why, when I was younger, I just hopped on the fast-food train like most everyone around me. I didn't know what I didn't know.

That's why I'm here, and you're reading this book. I'm like that little reminder on your shoulder wherever you go, whatever you do. ("What did that Dr. Healthnut dude say to eat or not eat?") Those former habits of mine have slowly changed over time. Twenty years ago, you couldn't force me to eat something healthy. Now, there's been a total transformation, coupled with the virtues of patience and pain. What? Pain a virtue? Well, to be honest, pain is the motivator for lifestyle metamorphosis. Eventually, the unhealthy food I was eating caused me a great deal of pain, motivating me to change my lifestyle. Healthnuts understand the critical importance of eating healthy and go to great *pains* to avoid unhealthy fast foods. And it's a lifelong experience. Although I've made some strides over the years, I am still learning every day.

THE THREE MAJOR DIETS

The three major diets are carbohydrate-focused diets, protein-focused di-ets, and fat-focused diets. You may find that now or at some point in your life you've tried one or even all of these with success or failure. Each have their own benefits and weaknesses. Keep in mind, a calorie is not just a calorie. As you read, be reminded that the *quality* of the calorie, and not just the quantity of calories, determine whether a carbohydrate, protein, or fat nutrient is unhealthy or healthy. I've provided several examples of diets that may work for each specific diet category.

CARBOHYDRATE-FOCUSED DIETS

CARBOHYDRATE DEMAND

Carbohydrate-focused diets are often a 70–20–10 split. When I say *split*, I mean the percentage of carbohydrates, proteins, and fats. Sometimes that's 70% carbohydrate, 20% protein, and 10% fat or 70% carbohydrate, 20% fat, and 10% protein. Other carb-focused diets are an 80–20 ratio with some combination of high carbs forming 80% of your diet while the other 20% is split between proteins and fats. For those high-carbohydrate diets that are healthier, some dieters attempt to overcome OB by using the 80–20 ratio.

Carbohydrates, after you eat them, break down into glucose. Glucose is properly transported into the cell when the pancreas releases the appropriate amount of insulin in response to the carbohydrate's conversion into glucose. The pancreas maintains blood sugar balance. During insulin resistance, there is a breakdown in the pancreas and in the body's ability to absorb and use glucose because the cells' insulin receptors are inhibited. The purpose of carbohydrates is to supply energy, like all food. Much of the reason for choosing carb-focused diets stems from the overconsumption of meats and fats because too much of the wrong meat and fat produces additional body stress and body toxicity.

GOOD CARBS?

Several high-carb diet books were released recently to bookstores everywhere. It's apparent that although high-carb diets were out of fashion in the last decade, they are now making a comeback. In the *The Starch Solution*, Dr. John McDougall makes the argument that starches themselves are not unhealthy. Rather, they are some of the most healthful foods. Starches include root vegetables such as tubers, potatoes, green vegetables, and other ground-based vegetables (complex carbs). Statistically, these diets show amazing results when it comes to reducing blood sugar, OB, and diseases of the heart. For example, studies demonstrate the positive cardiovascular, glucose

metabolism, and blood pressure effects of a high-carb diet, along with the beneficial nutrients like vitamin E, phytochemicals, and insoluble fiber as found
in whole grain brown rice.[36] Dr. McDougall has the evidence to back it up. His
clinical results with his patients are quite compelling and demonstrate reductions in all forms of chronic diseases.[37]

WRONG CARBS

Other high-carb diets reduce calories and center on the foods you probably enjoy. One of the challenges with these diets is that although they may
cause a short-term weight loss, you'll consume ingredients that may harm
other areas of your system. This is especially the case if the diet causes you to
consume carbohydrates that negatively impact insulin. Consuming fat-free,
carbohydrate-rich snacks will not help blood sugar balance. However, whole
foods that are high in micronutrients will.

For example, most whole fruits, like blueberries, pears, or apples, are negatively correlated with increasing the risk of type 2 diabetes. However, consuming fruit juices without the fiber, although very popular, are positively correlated with increased risk for type 2 diabetes. Ultimately, if not burned for
fuel, carbohydrates will be converted and stored as fat in the body. There is an
index that rates carbohydrates on their rate of conversion to glucose within the
human body, or their glycemic response—an important consideration.[38] This
index is called the glycemic index. (More on the glycemic index in chapter 15!)

RIGHT CARBS

The key to success with these plans is eating the right carbs and staying
off the wrong ones (simple carbs). In large scale studies as reported in *The
American Journal of Clinical Nutrition*, the quantity of carb-focused foods, like
fruits and vegetables, matters and is associated with a healthy heart.[39] There
is additional evidence, according to *JAMA*, that a higher intake of fruits and
vegetables and whole grains is very heart-healthy. Of course, this combination
must be coupled with healthy unsaturated fatty acids like omega-3. There is of
course still much debate on what ratio of carbs to fat translates to weight loss.[40]

Most high-carb diets that are successful eliminate sugar or other fat-
storing foods. You may even consider a carb-focused diet to be like vegetarian
diets—the difference being that a carb-focused diet may include some fats and
proteins, either vegetarian or animal-based.

HEALTHNUT CONS

- Carb diets that center on "healthy snacks" are not healthy because they contain simple carbs such as sugar, which your body quickly turns to fat.
- Carb diets may be protein and fat deficient if you're consuming mostly processed foods.
- Carb diets may increase health risk factors (cardiovascular disease, diabetes, etc.).

HEALTHNUT PROS

- Good carb diets may reduce health risk factors (cardiovascular disease, diabetes, etc.).
- Good carb diets may increase consumption of beneficial fiber (vegetables).
- Good carb diets may present weight reductions (if eating complex carbs).

PROTEIN-FOCUSED DIETS

EXTREME PROTEIN

Protein-focused diets can be as low as 30% protein to as high as 80% protein—or even higher! In this type of diet, the fats and carbohydrates are either moderately reduced or drastically reduced. The extremes of high-protein diets are sometimes followed by natural and professional body builders who consume inordinate amounts of protein and calories for periods of time to prepare for contests. Some of these practices may have arisen from animal studies that demonstrated that high-protein diets lead to fat reduction and improve glucose management.[41] Special event diets also drastically reduce the amount of carbs and increase protein before a show to "lean out."

When I followed a bodybuilding diet, I consumed a significant amount of the wrong "dead" proteins. Animal protein is often called "dead" protein. A "living" protein is plant-based and still contains its micronutrients. Once you heat any living protein over 100 degrees, it becomes a "dead" protein—meaning that it is denatured and loses its enzymes, etc., making it more difficult for the body to digest.

The overconsumption of dead proteins produced a high level of toxicity in my body. Immediately following this dietary lifestyle, I started having strange symptoms. In fact, one day I woke up from a nap with radiating chest pains at the tender age of twenty-one! Was this related to my high-protein diet? Possibly, but I cannot know for sure. What I do know is that the chest pains subsided after reducing my high-protein consumption.

Robert Atkins, MD, best-selling author of *The Atkins Diet*, is probably the most famous proponent of protein-focused diets. The best summarization of the now-deceased Dr. Atkins' life work is found in his *New York Times* best-seller, *Dr. Atkins' New Diet Revolution*. In the book, Dr. Atkins emphasizes very low carbohydrate consumption and very high-protein consumption, while at the same time reducing starches, including some high quality vegetables.[42] Higher protein intake has been shown to have a thermic effect as compared to higher carbohydrate or higher fat consumption. Animal protein tends to have a greater amino-acid composition profile versus some vegetarian forms. Protein also seems to give greater physiological and psycho-emotional satisfaction versus the other macronutrients.[43]

But the ubiquity of low-fat this and low-fat that all over our grocery stores begs the question: what changed over the last twenty years to make us dislike a high-protein diet? The change has to do, in part, with research done on high-protein dieters. One study of coronary heart disease risk, as reported in *Circulation*, spanning almost three decades and over 80,000 women, found that red meat consumption was associated with higher cardiovascular risk than poultry, fish, or low-fat dairy. However, it was difficult to discern the quality and sources of the meats used; there were plenty of foods like processed meats listed but whether there were also clean sources of meat with higher levels of beneficial fatty acids and other nutrients, is unknown. The study also detailed other negative lifestyle factors that were often associated with the red meat consumption.[44] According to *The American Journal of Clinical Nutrition*, diets too high in processed animal protein and red meat have been associated with type 2 diabetes and other cardiovascular risk factors.

However, it's important to note that higher protein has been correlated with weight loss and weight maintenance. As I mentioned before, I would like to suggest that the *quality* of the protein is more important than the *quantity*.

That's why, when replaced with chicken and fish, eggs, legumes, dairy, and nut sources of protein, the risk of high-protein diets decreases.[45] The most critical take-away from this discussion is that *quality matters!* More on this in part three!

PROTEIN + EXCESS = FAT

High-protein diets were the craze in the 1990s with several highly popularized athletes following them religiously. More recently, some researchers performed a significant analysis of dieting effectiveness and determined a carbohydrate-restricted diet with higher protein intake may be most effective in terms of weight loss.[46] What you are not told up front is that a very high-protein diet simply results in too much protein. And if you over-consume protein and your body does not use it, where does it go? Is it excreted? If it is, how much stress does that put on the organ processing all of that protein stored as fat?

It doesn't really matter whether the protein is from a healthy or an unhealthy source. Excess of any macronutrient is not beneficial. The body is smart. It takes only what is needed and either excretes or stores the rest. If your body determines that it is not nourished properly, it may begin to store the protein in your fat cells. This may manifest in different locations—some people have a tendency to store more belly fat or rear fat or even excessive organ fat.

A select group of genetically blessed people store fat and build muscle in all the right places—those few are what most of us would call freaks! I'm sure you've run across some of these in your lifetime; no matter what they eat or how little they exercise, they always seem to look healthy. But looks can be deceiving. Just because someone looks good on the outside does not necessarily mean they are healthy on the inside. Seriously, your body, not your wishful brain, determines how and where the fat gets stored. This is where your genetics play a small but important role in your health—although your own personal decisions play a much larger role.

A higher protein intake may provide a positive contribution to health in the case of athletes who have a larger protein requirement. They need more protein because they are constantly tearing down muscle tissue. This also depends on the specific athlete, type of sport, genetics, environmental influences, and stage of life. People ask me all the time which diet or lifestyle is the most effective. I hope that you are beginning to see why there is not just one simple dieting solution that works for everybody.

HEALTHNUT CONS

- Protein diets may increase risk for food intolerances and undigested proteins.
- Protein diets may increase health risk factors leading to autoimmune disease, cardiovascular disease, and cancer.
- Protein diets may tax the kidney, liver, and other excretory systems.

HEALTHNUT PROS

- Good protein diets may work for short-term weight loss and body fat reductions.
- Good protein diets may stabilize blood sugar and insulin imbalances.
- Good protein diets may be beneficial when increasing physical activity.

FAT-FOCUSED DIETS

FAT HEAD

Did you know that your neurological and brain system is composed of mostly fat? The brain is the largest fatty organ in the body! Fat used to be the bad guy in nutrition. But as pointed out in the journal *Experimental & Clinical Cardiology*, the OB culprit has switched from fat to the carbohydrate form of sugar—which can be stored as fat[47]—causing a renewed interest in fat-focused diets.

Fat-focused diets vary in the ratio of fat to other macronutrients: some recommend as low as 30% and some as high as 80% or more. High-fat diets may compliment high-protein diets to some degree. Ketogenic diets (which have higher levels of fat, moderate to high levels of protein, and low levels of carbohydrates) have been used in weight-loss therapies and shown to be effective, at least in the short term.[48] Depending on the type of fat consumed, the food selections will vary. Fats are utilized for long-term energy and storage in times of famine, and are found both in animal and vegetarian sources. Fats are also the ideal energy-burning tool for an efficient metabolism.

The right mix of fats is essential for a fat-focused diet. Sally Fallon heads the Weston Price Foundation that stands for real food, especially those that are of a fat source. Along with Dr. Mary Enig, Sally Fallon co-wrote *Eat Fat, Lose Fat*. The authors describe the health and weight-loss benefits of a high-fat diet especially consisting of coconut oil.[49] Some people increase the right types of fat nutrients, such as coconut oil, to support fat burning.

Keep in mind, however, that there are also unhealthy fats that are detrimental to humans, just like there are unhealthy carbohydrates and proteins that are also detrimental. Let me give you an example.

Don't eat too many nuts! I would tell myself before a nightly binge on nuts. When I traveled for business and stayed often in hotels, I would get unlimited, free roasted and salted nuts—one of the perks of being on the road three weeks out of each month. However, those nuts were fried in unhealthy vegetable oils. The salt was like a dry ice that arrested my cardiovascular and digestive systems and kept me up all night. Seriously, I would eat so many, I'd end up with a bloated stomach. I'd tell myself *never again*, but I just couldn't resist that addictive salty taste—and the fact that they were free. The next night, I'd reward myself by binging yet again!

I finally came to realize that I was consuming the wrong, unhealthily transformed version of nuts. Nuts, in the right form and full of fat, are actually healthy! In epidemiological studies, the unsaturated fat in nuts is heart-healthy, contains beneficial minerals like magnesium, nutrients like vitamin E, beneficial fiber, and potassium.[50] Compare this to saturated animal fat (yes, that disgusting, glue-like substance that hangs off the slab of beef). Regardless of where you land on the nutritional belief spectrum, it seems self-evident that we were not meant to consume saturated animal fat in large amounts. To be fair, I am not necessarily saying that all animal fat is bad for everyone. Some believe that healthy, grass-fed sources of fat-filled animal glands like beef liver are loaded with beneficial vitamins and nutrients. The vegetarian version of beneficial fats would be coconut oil.

Healthier fats, even in moderate amounts, are associated with a reduction in lifestyle diseases and OB risk factors such as visceral fat, insulin resistance, and inflammation, as discussed in *The New England Journal of Medicine*.[51]

FAT ENERGY

Some sports do require considerable energy stores and may require an increased fat intake. Some climates may also require additional fat in the diet. For example, Alaskans traditionally consume a high amount of fatty fish or even other odd delicacies that enables their bodies to endure their climate's grueling winters.

They may have also been getting essential micronutrients from their diet. I worked with a practitioner that used to joke about his consumption of whale blubber. That was a big thing a few years ago! The real benefit of the fat is found in the key fat-soluble vitamins—A, D, E, and K. My practitioner friend likely recommended the whale fat to his patients because he knew it was almost impossible to over-consume fat-soluble vitamins when they are packaged in a food source like blubber. On the other hand, obtaining these vitamins from a gel cap or pill does open you up to the potential toxicity of over-consumption.

Won't increasing fat intake lead to disease and more body fat? Interestingly, the times I've consumed a 50% or higher fat diet, I've actually been at what I consider my perfect weight. Again, I was consuming the right fats and not the wrong ones! Remember, numerous studies reveal that higher body fat content is associated with a risk of many degenerative diseases. Do those diseases occur from consuming all fats or just some fats? Do some fats protect your body from degenerative diseases? For example, DHA, the essential fatty acid associated with reducing the risk of cardiovascular disease, is found in lower concentrations in those who struggle with OB.[52]

FAT + LESS = LONGEVITY

Other studies show longevity correlates with consuming less fat and calories as a whole. In the mid-twentieth century, most of the American population ate a larger percentage of fat to their total caloric intake than most twenty-first-century Americans do.[53] And yet, a larger percentage of the US population today has heart disease and other OB-related conditions than a century ago. From this we can see that eating fat may not necessarily correlate to stored and harmful fatty deposits in your cardiovascular system. The amount of storage (which evidences itself in extra pounds on your body) depends on the type of fat and on your particular biology.

HEALTHNUT CONS

- Inflammatory fat diets may increase health-risk factors (because of hydrogenated fats, etc.).
- Fat diets may decrease life span when the fat is stored as visceral or organ fat.
- Fat diets may lack fiber and contribute to digestive difficulties.

HEALTHNUT PROS

- Good anti-inflammatory fat diets may burn body fat and reduce health-risk factors.
- Good fat diets may increase essential fat-soluble vitamins and minerals.
- Good fat diets may be vital in critical seasons, such as pregnancy or intense activity.

I think you see the trend here as I review these diet types—there is no one-size-fits-all diet. However, all successful diets may have one thing in common. In a large-scale study (meta-analysis) of adults aged 18–70 regarding their dietary macronutrient intake, researchers found it was not the ratio percentage of carbohydrates, proteins, and fats that mattered as much as it was the quality of nutrients. For example, increasing fiber-rich foods and reducing low quality foods like sugar were a higher determinant of whether participants found weight-loss success.[54] Long-term success, it appears, depends on whether the food is healthy, not on whether it's a carbohydrate, fat, or protein.

HEALTHNUT POPULAR

T he three most popular diets are vegetarian diets, fasting diets, and metabolism diets. Are there other popular diets? Absolutely, but these three diet themes are the most prevalent worldwide. Some of these diets are used for a lifetime while others are designed to be implemented periodically—such as fasting. Within each of the diets are, of course, many sub-diets. Most important, remember that just because a diet is popular does not necessarily mean it is right for you.

VEGETARIAN DIETS

VEGETARIAN MEDLEY DIETS

Vegetarian diets, like carb-focused diets, are often a 70–20–10 macronutrient combination, with 70% carbohydrates, 20% protein, 10% fat. However, this ratio may vary and have higher or lower concentrations of vegetarian-based fat or protein. The difference between vegetarian and carb-focused diets is that vegetarian diets are made up exclusively of plant sources.

Although vegetarian diets do not include any animal products, occasionally excepting limited quantities of eggs and fish or, in some cases, animal products from honey and dairy, they usually do include a balance of macronutrients because of their wide variety of food combinations. This is possible because the amino acids in fruits and vegetables vary hugely, and one can gain nutrient density by eating a large enough variety.

Distinguished Cornell University nutrition professor T. Colin Campbell is famous for his work in *The China Study*. The conclusion of this exhaustive compilation of evidence is that vegetarian diets with a reduction of processed foods virtually eliminate the chronic diseases of our modern culture.[55] As reported in the *Nutrition Journal*, other large scale studies from Seventh-Day Adventists and Indian vegetarians report protection against hypertension and type 2 diabetes, often through foods that have a lower glycemic index such as some whole grains, legumes, nuts, beans, and vegetables, to reduce chronic inflammation and oxidative stress.[56] Although Dr. Campbell admits that integrating a vegetarian diet into every facet of life is controversial, his data indicates that a diet in unrefined plant foods (while reducing fat, salt, and sugar) convincingly heals chronic disease.[57]

There has been a definite trend and a movement toward more vegetarian and vegan type diets in the last several years. Some of this is sparked by our culture's over-consumption of unhealthy animal proteins and fats. Others are concerned about the rights of animals and follow the diet for political or environmental purposes. I received a recent social media message claiming that vegetarian is the only conscionable diet for humanitarian and health considerations. In the US, vegetarian diets are becoming more socially acceptable. Restaurants are offering more vegetarian options for people. There is a string of strict vegetarian restaurants popping up all over the country as well. In the US, much of this revolutionary movement stems from California and New York.

When I tried the strict vegetarian diet, I found that initially I had tremendous energy, and my liver healed from years of toxic buildup. Consistent with the benefits that meta-analysis of vegetarian diets have demonstrated, my cardiovascular system, blood pressure, and lipid levels all improved![58] There was one side effect that many people would love, but I didn't: I lost weight. That was not my goal! (But actually, I don't know many true vegetarians who struggle with OB. Is that a coincidence?) However, I needed to incorporate this type of eating plan, at least temporarily, because I was consuming so much unhealthy animal products and processed foods. The diet was a complete 180-degree turn in my diet from vegetarian deficiency to vegetarian extreme. In some cases, like mine, extremely negative habits may require extreme, temporary remedies.

Over time, however, I was increasingly fatigued throughout the day. So I added a little animal protein (specifically fish) back into my diet and felt more energized. Some vegetarians will include eggs, milk, and even fish into their diets. Fish is considered a special kind of meat because it is water-based versus land-based. Some fish have high omega-3 fatty acids that are beneficial for joints, brain, and nervous system function. Back when I was a kid, I never really liked fish. Thankfully, tastes change over the years! In my opinion, fish is the perfect animal food. However, the rise of toxic element contamination from the environment and our ecosystem can make seafood consumption more dangerous (see chapter 15 for more information).

Some healthnuts I've consulted with want to stay with a vegetarian life-style while others switch back to animal. Still others go back and forth be-tween animal- and plant-based diets depending on their season in life and the level of activity required of them on a day-to-day basis.

I think the success with a vegetarian diet is intimately connected to one's culture, genetic and familial history, purpose in life, and overall health. I've seen some vegetarian diets that are extremely unhealthy because they're full of high-sodium packaged and processed foods. They may include unhealthy forms of soy that are actually anti-nutrients instead of other forms of soy, such as fermented versions, that are a much better choice.[59] However, I've seen other vegetarian meal plans that are quite healthy and deliciously balanced.

VEGAN DIETS

The second main type of vegetarian diet is the vegan diet. There are dif-ferent vegan diets but primarily vegans eliminate both cooked and raw animal foods, all dairy, and all eggs. However, they include cooked vegetarian foods such as vegan soups as long as they do not contain any dairy or eggs.

Although this is a trend in the US, you'll be surprised to discover that a Gallup poll conducted within the last several years found only 5% of the popu-lation considered themselves vegetarian and only 2% would call themselves vegan.[60] Interestingly, vegan diets especially benefit males.[61] There are some downsides because vegans may have more of a challenge with acquiring suffi-cient amounts of vitamin B12, calcium, and protein, compared to non-vegans.

Dr. Joel Fuhrman, author of the *New York Times* best seller *Eat to Live*, is one of the foremost authorities on a plant-based vegan diet. In his book, Dr. Fuhrman claims that the healthiest foods are living foods. Instead of pro-cessed foods and dairy and meat products, he advocates a stringent, nutrient-dense diet of whole foods including vegetables, fruits, legumes, seeds, and nuts.[62] I've had the privilege of meeting with Dr. Fuhrman and I can tell you he is very passionate about nutrition and health—also evidenced in the many successes he's had with his patients.

Dr. Fuhrman may be the first to admit that vegan diets are one of the strictest of the vegetarian diets. However, I don't think he believes that's to a dieter's detriment. But because vegans eliminate all eggs, cheese, milk, and target specific plant-based foods, it may be more difficult to get protein with these diets unless carefully planned out. Other experts, similar to Dr. Fuhrman, believe we don't need as much protein in our diets as we've been told.

Many people lose weight on these diets but other healthcare experts argue that vegan diets may create other deficiencies over the long term. However, there are aspects to vegan diets, at least practiced in the short term, that can add tremendous health benefits by reducing stress and fighting disease. It is reported that the gut microbiome of vegans is supportive for reducing inflammation, metabolic syndrome, and OB, because of the increase of plant food sources and—especially—fiber (fiber can help feed beneficial bacteria). With the increase of these compounds in the diet, there appears to be a better gut protection mechanism. Many vegans also consume more nutrient-dense foods that are healthier than traditional, processed foods.[63] But if you are a vegan who does not eat enough healthy food, your body won't react well. Again, it seems to boil down to a question of the *quality* of your consumption!

If you ask some of the most famous centenarians in the US, you'll find many of these hundred-year-olds, and older, live in Loma Linda, California. Loma Linda is considered one of the longest-lived hotspot regions of the world along with Okinawa, Japan, and areas of Ecuador, Italy, and Greece, collectively referred to as the Blue Zones. Many of the local Loma Linda population consume mostly a vegan and vegetarian diet. Most of the zones follow principles of eating slowly, eating mostly plants, and eating smaller sized meals as the day moves on.[64] This equates to less chronic disease on the whole compared to other population groups. This sounds incredible, right? These inhabitants of the Blue Zones hold the secret to aging well!

Before you get too excited, however, some detractors who participated in a vegan diet found an increased propensity to chronic diseases, perhaps because they were eating the wrong type of vegan foods, not supplementing their diet, or not eating the healthy ratio of micronutrients to macronutrients. Also note that at least one of the Blue Zones includes animal-based meat and dairy.[65] It appears that health outcomes are related to not just *what* macronutrient we consume, but also the ratio of which we consume it!

LACTO-OVO DIETS

Lacto-ovo is a vegetarian diet that includes eggs and milk. However, it must be the right type of eggs or milk and not the standard processed eggs and milk products found in most supermarkets. This diet differs from the lacto-vegetarian which includes only milk products and vegetables, or the ovo-vegetarian which only includes eggs and vegetables. Each of these diets excludes meat, seafood, and poultry.[66]

The concern with some of the vegan diets that exclude dairy and eggs is their impact on bone mineral density over the long term. The elderly are often victim to fractures that leave them in a hospital setting where they are at risk for contracting some pathogen, bacteria, or virus that eventually leads to death. Some concerned with bone health adopt milk and/or eggs into their vegetarian diet. In some small studies, it is reported that there is no bone loss associated with these variations of the vegetarian diet in young people. I have no doubt that this will be confirmed in larger studies in the future.[67]

Others, however, may be allergic to either milk or eggs, causing them to exclude them from their diet. It is absolutely vital to find out what foods you are intolerant of or allergic to so these foods do not act as an anti-nutrient in your body (an anti-nutrient is a natural or synthetic compound that blocks or inhibits the body's normal absorption of nutrients).

MACROBIOTIC DIETS

For practical reasons, macrobiotic diets are usually a specialty, short-term vegetarian diet used to cleanse or heal the digestive system. Several Asian cultures incorporate a macrobiotic approach to their meals, either in combination with other foods or as the main dish. Macrobiotic diets consist mostly of liquid vegetarian meals such as healing soups. The original macrobiotic diets were derived from ancient eastern philosophy to provide healing for gut or metabolic disorders. An example of a macronutrient ratio is 50% whole grains, 40% vegetables, and 10% legumes. Additional micronutrient-based fermented foods, such as miso for its probiotic effect or mineral-dense seaweed are also included, along with healing teas. These particular diets often eliminate all animal products, eggs, dairy, any additional sugars, and all processed foods.[68]

In some studies, blood glucose levels improved substantially in type 2 diabetic patients in as little as twenty-one days on a macrobiotic diet.[69] Although the research done on macrobiotic diets is far more limited than the amount of research done on other well-known diets, the speed at which healing occurs in this diet promises to outperform metabolic healing in other vegetarian, fasting, or metabolic diets.

FIBER DIETS

Dietary fiber is a complex carbohydrate with many different synergistic factors that may provide beneficial bacterial fermentation, and that resists digestion and absorption into the small intestines.[70] Dr. Denis Burkit popularized the idea that fiber protects against lifestyle diseases including OB. As we begin to understand more about the importance of the microbiota and health, we are beginning to learn more about the fibrous prebiotics which support the GI tract via fermentation of microflora to stimulate the growth and well-being of beneficial bacteria or probiotics in the gut.[71]

The benefits of fiber may include reduced risk factors of metabolic syndrome, cardiovascular disease, and inflammatory processes. Fiber also provides a sense of fullness, which contributes to a healthy weight. Although there are many benefits to increasing the amount of fiber, the SAD diet is regrettably void of fibers, both in their soluble form (oats, legumes, barley, fruits, and vegetables) and their insoluble form (bran and cereal grains).[72]

Fiber diets are arranged for a cleansing of the large and small intestines, restoring healthy bowel function, removing toxins, increasing healthy blood flow, and balancing blood sugar. A popular form of fiber diet is to use fruits and vegetables in soups, beverages, or eaten raw and whole. Other fiber diets may include whole grains, but this may or may not be as effective as the fruit and vegetable-based fibers. Just be careful to avoid consuming too much fiber, though, as it will cause loose stools and possibly other unpleasant odors.

RAW FOOD DIETS

Raw food diets are the extreme of pure vegan dieting. Raw foodists remove not only animal protein but all cooked foods, including cooked vegetarian foods. Some raw food diets attempt to make the body more alkaline by removing the more acidic animal foods and replacing them with leafy green plants, whether in juice or whole food form, based on the theory that the more alkalinity your blood has, the less disease it has. A pH scale, or potential hydrogen scale, divides your body's fluid balance between the high numbers of alkaline and the low numbers of acidic. However, health is not solely limited to pH balance within the body.

Now, in some instances, raw diets produce a vibrancy of health. An example of this is found in boosting the intake of the antioxidants, phytochemicals, and beneficial fibers found in raw fruits, vegetables, nuts, and seeds. There is a broad level of research that indicates the benefits of these nutrients that range from lowering cancer risk to weight reduction.[73] I've never met a single raw foodist who appeared to struggle with OB—but as we've discussed, the external is not the only determinant of health. In other instances, participants suffer from pathogenic infections from bacteria-laden foods. The raw diets may even overlap with fasting diets. Some choose to stay on the raw diet long term.

In my observations with some healthnuts, there is a danger of being deficient in some nutrients that your body needs if you opt for 100% raw. For example, it's known that some raw green leafy vegetables have lower levels of antioxidants than when cooked. Similarly, nutrients from tomatoes are more available to your body when cooked compared to raw.[74] That's probably why many people opt to choose a combination of high raw with some cooked. Besides, unless you live in one of those perfect, sunny climates year round, those cold winter nights can be quite chilling without some warm, delicious, vegan soup! However, I want to make it clear that a raw diet may be very beneficial for at least a period of time or under specific circumstances.

HEALTHNUT CONS

- Vegetarian diets without adequate protein may cause muscle atrophy.
- Vegetarian diets may create inflammation by eating processed vegetarian foods.
- Vegetarian diets may cause deficiencies in fat-soluble vitamins B12, D, K, E, and A.

HEALTHNUT PROS

- Good vegetarian diets may improve cardiovascular health, blood sugar, and OB.
- Good vegetarian diets may increase energy, clear inflammation, and cause healing.
- Good vegetarian diets provide a variety of food for adequate protein and nutrients.

FASTING DIETS

In basic terms, fasting is limiting or going without food or even drink for periods of time. Fasting diets may also include giving up different types of foods for an extended or indefinite timeframe. Based on research from both animal and human studies, fasting has been shown to have beneficial protective effects when dealing with hypertension, metabolic syndrome, neurodegeneration, cancer, aging, and especially OB. A standard range of fasting is from a half day up to twenty-one days and may include sacrifices of both food and high-caloric beverages (but not fasting from water—water is vital).[75] Research on both humans and animals has found weight-loss success from these caloric reductions or periodic fasts.[76]

Fasting can also be done for spiritual reasons in addition to physical purposes, like the Daniel Fast.[77] The Daniel Fast, which lasts from anywhere between 10 and 21 days, is a fast from any choice foods such as meat, wine, sugar, or any other refined or processed foods. The real focus is to become closer to God through prayer, meditation, and scriptural readings that accompany the physical aspects of the fast.[78]

If you've struggled with OB, fasting diets can either be good or bad: If done improperly, fasting diets can actually cause a person to store more fat and weight. If done properly, they can also cause a person to utilize more of the stored body fat. Some types of fasting are for life, while others are for as little as a few hours to days to weeks to even months.

Some of the most popular food fasting diets include eating whole foods— such as vegetables or fruits—while giving up protein and fats. They can either be raw food fasts or even cooked fasts. The benefits of whole food fasting are primarily the increase of fiber and colon cleansing properties. Consuming an increase of fruits and vegetables allows for the food and especially the fiber to bind to and remove toxins out of your system. Although these fasts may be beneficial, they are not as healing as vegetable juice fasts, for example.

And then there is extreme fasting—no food at all for long periods of time. I read of someone who tried an air fasting diet. There's another word for prolonged air fasting—starvation! It's not something I would recommend.

INTERMITTENT FASTING

As reported in the *Nutrition Journal*, intermittent fasting along with alternate-day fasts have been shown in small clinical trials to be effective for moderate weight loss, fat loss, and waist circumference reductions within short periods of time.[79] Dr. Michael Mosley is the author of the best seller *The Fast Diet*. Although there are many types of fasting diets, Mosley describes the simplicity of cutting out a few days' worth of excess calories by limiting two days each week to only 500 calories per day.[80] What this equates to is reducing your diet by 1000 calories per week. There are about 3500 calories per pound of body weight, so by eating 1000 fewer calories per week, you lose at least several pounds per month.

Dr. Mosley's message is pretty simple, targeting those who have the last ten to twenty pounds to lose. You fast at least eight out of thirty days per month and you'll lose those extra pounds automatically. There appears to be little if any side effects in terms of energy, sleep, or GI disruptions during alternative fasting days.[81]

JUICE FASTING

Juice fasting, a fast where all food consumed is juiced, is healing for the intestinal track and other organs because it provides the body a break from digestion. Juice fasting may be a fast by itself or it may be used in combination with other types of foods. There are several juice fasting variations. The main fasts are vegetable juice fasting, which may be more insulin-friendly, or fruit juice fasting. Fruit juice fasting may cause a rise in blood sugar, even with the cleansing properties, depending on whether the juice contains the fiber or not.

It is well-established that diets comprised of plenty of fruits and vegetables are weight-friendly and reduce the risk of lifestyle diseases.[82] Juicing is one of the easiest methods to receive a wide variety of vegetables and fruits with rapid uptake into the bloodstream. There are research observations that demonstrate a simple addition of vegetable juice caused participants to lose more weight compared to those who did not consume vegetable juice. What is most surprising to me is this was not freshly pressed, but juice from a can![83] How much more effective would fresh vegetable juice demonstrate to be if it were compared in a clinical trial?

Overall, I want to make absolutely clear that, from an OB perspective, a juice fast under appropriate holistic healthcare approval and supervision may provide significant health and weight benefits over a brief or extended period of time. A properly supervised juice fast may last for, 7, 21, 30, 60, or even 90 days or more!

HEALTHNUT CONS

- Water fasting may be hard on the body but still lead to major healing (ask your physician before trying).
- Fruit juice fasting without fiber may contain too much sugar (ask your physician before trying).
- Juice fasting may be dangerous if prolonged (ask your physician before trying).

HEALTHNUT PROS

- Vegetable juice fasting is primarily used to create alkalinity in the body.
- Vegetable juice fasting is rapidly assimilated into the bloodstream, providing healing to digestive organs.
- Fruit juice fasting that contains fiber is primarily cleansing.

DETOXIFICATION DIETS

Detox diets have also become very popular. Some healthnuts use the term *purification* instead of detox, but they are really one and the same. (Don't confuse a detox diet with detoxing from substance abuse, such as a drug or alcohol detox.) Detox diets assume that you are consuming "toxins" and often recommend individually or collectively removing foods like unhealthy grains, meats, all sugar and caffeine, and other highly addictive and processed foods. How successful are these diets? Some work great! Others have questionable evidence on how effectively they "remove" toxins.

Dr. Alejandro Junger, the *New York Times* best-selling author of *Clean*, believes that a detoxification approach to health is the best approach. Much of his book centers on smoothies and liquid nutrition and eliminating harmful foods.[84] There are also recommended supplements. Some physicians feel that dietary supplements are not necessary. Other physicians believe evidence-based nutritional supplements are a critical part of the process for reducing cravings. The reality is that supplements are not necessary if you consume the fresh raw herbs to do what the supplements are intended to accomplish—and how many people are actually going to do that?

DETOX DILEMMA

Get rid of the bad and eat the good. That's what detoxing is really about. It's a nice term for a modified elimination diet and is really the sibling to fasting diets. The difference, however, is that detoxification often requires caloric intake, because fasting from all foods may cause redistribution of toxic accumulation in the body (especially if consuming powerful herbs or dietary supplements). Does it work? Sure it can work. However, *which* type of detox will work for you is a whole different question.

I met with a practitioner one time to consult on growing her weight-loss practice. One of the elements she was lacking in her practice was a detoxification protocol for her patients. She took her patients directly into the weight-loss program without first preparing the body for the weight-loss process. But if her patient's elimination and metabolic systems were not optimal, which can be accomplished through a careful detox to help the liver and other organs work more optimally, the weight loss could be more time-consuming.

When I started to suggest that detoxing would help her patients, she got really upset. "Detox! Do you know how many people have died from that?" she exclaimed. Of course, she didn't understand that it was a nutritional detox. She, like many in the medical community, was reluctant to embrace effective nutritional therapies. Thankfully, this mind-set is shifting with the influx of integrative-minded, lifestyle, holistic physicians.

On my way out of her office, I caught a glimpse of the weight-loss products she offered to her patients. Although some of her patients were losing an effective amount of weight, the products she peddled were horrible in terms of nutritional quality. The patients were consuming fewer calories, but those calories were full of fake food ingredients with limited nutritional benefit. It's easy to see that these patients lost weight by simply consuming fewer calories, while at the same time accumulating nutritional "toxicity." This toxicity may come back to bite them later, post weight-loss.

DETOX DECISIONS

Recommended detox periods vary. Some are a 3-day detox, some 7-day, 21-day, 30-day, or even longer! Some healthnuts do detox diets with the seasons of the year. (Of course, Floridians really only have two seasons, so compared to the north they are getting two less detoxes per year!) Other healthnuts do a continual detox, but those diets tend to be more challenging to maintain over the long term.

Animal-product detox diets include food such as meat, eggs, and dairy as part of the process. Many claim that during detox there is still a need to support the system with animal-based nutrients. If you take food away, the fast may release more toxins throughout your body or even redeposit those toxins somewhere else in the body! This theory also claims that detoxing is so hard on the system, some proteins and fats are necessary. Many practitioners I consult use the animal form of detox.

Plant detox diets, on the other hand, are more closely aligned with fasting. Plant detox dieting eliminates the stress of animal foods. It's very important to only participate in this detox—or any detox—with a holistic health care professional experienced with nutritional therapies. Detox may stress your body so it's important to not just jump in, but to effectively prepare the body for a detox.

HEALTHNUT CONS

- Detox programs, even good detox programs, may cause harm if done improperly.
- Detox programs may release toxins too rapidly and either redistribute the toxins or stress the body.
- Detox programs with inferior dietary supplements may harm the body.

HEALTHNUT PROS

- Good detox programs may rejuvenate the liver, kidneys, digestive, and other organs.
- Good detox programs may help you eliminate difficult to remove symptoms.
- Good detox program benefits vary depending on the type of detox.

CRON

Another specific type of fasting diet is Calorie Restriction Optimal Nutrition (CRON). UCLA professor Dr. Roy Walford is the pioneer behind calorie restriction while utilizing optimal nutrition. For over seventy years, he hypothesized that caloric restriction slows the aging process (although just before his death in 2004, he did admit that more studies would be required to validate CRON's findings). The initial research hints at a positive step toward understanding human mortality.[85]

CRON reduces the amount of calories while maximizing the nutrients that flood your cells with living fuel. It maintains the same meal frequency schedule throughout the day, but reduces the amount of calories and increases the amount of nutrients, in this way differing from general fasting.[86] In a nutshell, the CRON theory is that those who consume the least amount of calories live the longest. This is especially found in those who are centenarians. Overall, centenarians tend to eat less but have higher consumption yields of nutrients. However, that doesn't mean that they ate this way their whole lives; usually it was later in life that they took a calorie-restricted approach. Such an approach would not be appropriate, for example, for someone who is in child-bearing years where extra healthful calories may be vitally important. Without the proper amounts of nutrient-dense foods such as healthy fats and proteins, it is more challenging to keep hormones and neurotransmitters and brain chemicals optimal. The latter three are heavily tied to gastrointestinal health as well.

LESS IS MORE

If you analyze CRON just by nature of caloric intake, it is more carbohydrate-intensive and has fewer dense foods, such as proteins and fats. The CRON diet adheres to the principle that it is important to burn more calories than you eat. In the US, we tend to consume more food than we burn. Our unhealthy food portion sizes are often out of control, especially when you consider that the food is usually unhealthy! Remember that real, healthy, food may be consumed in unlimited amounts when the body is properly balanced. You'll know when you've had enough, and you naturally won't desire to overindulge.

Overconsumption is one of the main contributors to the OB epidemic. If we either consume fewer unhealthy calories or participate in some form of moderate ongoing activity, we will most likely experience a healthy weight, and even a maximized life span.[87] In studies done on animals, restricting calories by as much as 50% included additional benefits such as protection against lifestyle and chronic diseases.[88] The other advantage of CRON is that dieters typically receive higher quality nutrition that fuels the cells.

Although I often see CRON diet favored among those more advanced in years, the growing trend is for young people to abstain from foods as well, especially in the form of a vegan diet. Vegans push for longevity by maximizing nutrient quality versus caloric intake. It's important to note that a CRON diet demonstrates longevity in mice, but it may cause other yet-unidentified deficiencies in humans in the long-term. Overall, unless there are unique dietary needs, consuming higher nutrient foods and fewer nutrient-deficient foods relates to more energy and a higher quality of life.

HEALTHNUT CONS

- CRON diets may be deficient in some nutrients.
- CRON diets may only work during certain life phases.
- CRON diets may be somewhat limited in variety.

HEALTHNUT PROS

- CRON diets are associated with longer lived populations.
- CRON diets may provide a high quality of life with dense food reductions.
- CRON diets center on quality of nutrition versus quantity.

METABOLISM DIETS

Boosting the metabolism, which is the real key to eliminating OB, and inflammation go hand in hand. If you peruse the literature and popular press, many of the weight-loss advocates push for some variation of reducing systemic inflammation. I am not talking about reducing all inflammation; after all, it can be an essential warning sign when things just aren't going well! The word *inflammation* is often thrown around like it's the enemy. And yes, it is the enemy when it gets out of control and causes autoimmune inflammatory reactions that cannot be controlled and lead to lifestyle diseases. However, during normal body function, we want some level of inflammation for protection and healing. In terms of diet, we don't want the systemic inflammation with body dysfunction. This is why a balanced view of reducing the negative inflammation through a healthy diet is so popular.

The main benefits in the metabolic philosophy leads to a metabolism-boosting, energy-supplying, blood-sugar-balancing, cardiovascular-supporting, and heart-healthy lifestyle. Yet one metabolic diet may include more whole grains and carbs (such as Mediterranean) while another (such as paleo) limits grains and carbs in general. One is more plant-based with the exception of fish and reducing saturated fats (Mediterranean) while the other may be generally more animal or a combination of animal and plant with more saturated fats (again, paleo). Both diets promote avoiding processed and refined foods, sugar, and reducing or eliminating dairy. But, as always, there are also detractors who believe too many whole grains, higher fats from oils, or fish in the traditional Mediterranean diets or higher amounts of animal proteins and fats from nuts in the paleo diets can lead to OB and other forms of toxicity.

MEDITERRANEAN DIET

The Mediterranean diet get its fame from the fact that this traditional dietary pattern is based on the traditional lifestyle patterns of those living around the Mediterranean Sea. Although there is variation among the cultural interpretation of the Mediterranean dietary theme, most share common characteristics. Traditional Mediterranean eating patterns include an abundance of fruits and vegetables, a higher intake of fats especially from monounsaturated sources such as olive oil, and high vegetable protein such as legumes and nuts. Some may include a high amount of fish but are lower in other forms of land animal-based protein.[89] Personally, I've eaten at "Mediterranean" restaurants that include turkey, chicken, lamb, and other clean meats, so it's debatable whether this is the modernized version of the Mediterranean or traditional Mediterranean.

Large population studies as described in the *British Medical Journal* report overall lower mortality, lower cancer mortality and incidence, and reduced risk of Alzheimer's or Parkinson's from the traditional aspects of the Mediterranean diets.[90] Outside of external environmental factors, many Mediterranean population groups tend to not have the degenerative diseases that western cultures struggle with. They have one of the lowest incidences of these lifestyle diseases of all population groups. Is this all related to diet and lifestyle? To a large extent, yes. Do they have any less stress? Not necessarily. However, their lifestyles and diets almost override the negative stress from their external environment. These observations led many to institute diets based on what these population groups normally eat.

Keep in mind there are variations of Mediterranean diets although they all follow the same theme. There is an ample amount of research that Mediterranean-based diets are heart-healthy and longevity-enhancing. Some people say it's because of the polyphenolic resveratrol in red wine. In my estimation, there is much more going on than just the red wine. Benefits include a lower risk of cardiovascular disease, inflammation, less LDL oxidation, increased weight loss, and lower blood pressure. For those population groups who consume a higher fish intake, there is increased omega-3 fatty acid consumption that lowers the risk of cardiac deaths and increases vascular function. According to *The American Journal of Clinical Nutrition*, those who increase their level of fiber from whole grains, vegetables, fruits, nuts, legumes benefit from weight reductions, glucose metabolism, and unhealthy lipid level decreases.[91]

The Mediterranean diet is often full of balanced macronutrients and micronutrients, usually on a 40–30–30 macronutrient ratio. Whether the order is carbs, proteins, and fats or proteins, carbs, and fats, the ratio may adjust. The Mediterranean diet tends to be more balanced than other diets and reduces the amount of inflammation for many people. The diet usually contains an ample amount of fish, vegetables, whole grains, and fiber.

Some studies link longevity to eating fatty fish with omega-3s every week.[92] Yet an article from the *New York Times* reports that in Mediterranean cultures, at least half the population is overweight in Italy, Portugal, and

Spain.[93] This makes for an interesting discussion. Why do the people that live in the Mediterranean have these incidents of OB? Or how about people on this side of the ocean: what's our definition of Mediterranean? A huge plate of spaghetti for dinner may appear Mediterranean, but it's not authentic. Are we really consuming an optimal Mediterranean diet or a modified processed diet that has the Mediterranean label on it? Studies continue to support the claim that *traditional* Mediterranean diets are effective for preventing OB-related issues.[94]

HEALTHNUT CONS

- Mediterranean diets may favor one macronutrient over another.
- Mediterranean diets may support weight-promoting, unhealthy foods.
- Present-day Mediterranean cultures have increased OB issues (possibly due to adoption of SAD).

HEALTHNUT PROS

- Mediterranean diets provide a balanced macronutrient approach.
- Mediterranean diets may support a healthy heart and reduce chronic inflammation.
- Mediterranean diets provide beneficial essential fatty acids, antioxidants, and phenolics.

There are subsets of this diet that limit whole grains that I'll discuss in the next section.

PALEOLITHIC DIET

The paleolithic diet, or paleo, is a specific type of metabolism diet. Paleo is based on an approximation of what our human ancestors would have consumed—hence the name, "paleolithic"—such as lean meats, seeds, nuts, vegetables, fruits, and healthy fats. It excludes refined sugar, processed oils, salt, dairy, legumes, and grains. It's also often referred to as a hunter-gatherer, Stone Age, or caveman diet. Proponents that believe this diet predates the introduction of agricultural products like grains, which made an appearance relatively recently. Observationally, paleo proponents believe this diet prevents obesity and metabolic syndrome. There is especially a call for additional research regarding the long term effects regarding this diet's high vitamin D levels, calcium, and potential toxicity with mercury from fish consumption.[95]

For example, the modernized version of the Mediterranean diet may include a higher amount of land animal proteins and less whole grains compared to traditional Mediterranean diets with more whole grains and limited to no animal protein (except fish). Keep in mind there are emotional and psychosocial factors in diet consumption. In one analysis, the paleo diet with lean meat, fish, nuts, vegetables, eggs, and fruits, was more satisfying to dieters than a high-grain, low-fat dairy, fish, fruit, and vegetable-based Mediterranean diet.[96]

The paleo diet shares with the Mediterranean diet the purpose of eliminating inflammation by removing potentially inflammatory foods (even if they differ on which foods those include). Paleo may remove inflammatory grains and specifically gluten or even dairy. Yet there is some blend between the diets even if the literature does not always acknowledge it. For example, although two paleo dietary traditions contain a large amount of protein and fats from animal and plant sources, one paleo tradition comes from the Mediterranean region and more closely resembles the traditional Mediterranean ratios. You can see why anti-inflammation or metabolic diets have a wide variety of perspectives!

Paleo certainly shares the abundance of vegetables, fruits, healthy fats, and nuts with traditional Mediterranean. In a two-year trial of OB women published in the *European Journal of Clinical Nutrition*, the paleo diet, with its increase of protein, increase of unsaturated fats, and reduction of carbohydrates, had positive effects on fat mass, abdominal obesity, and triglyceride levels as compared to a low-fat and high-fiber diet, although larger scale clinical trials are needed to confirm these findings.[97]

Paleo is different from plant diets because one consumes more proteins and fats, which may also include abundant animal sources. For example, the diet eliminates most grains, with the exception of flax seeds, on the predication that our ancestors ate a diet devoid of grains. Some healthnuts that are on a gluten-free diet will often go paleo. The reason for this switch is their inability to properly assimilate the pro-inflammatory protein, gluten. Gluten may cause systemic inflammation through the GI tract and this can be verified through specific immune testing. Paleo eases your GI tract because it contains no gluten at all. Paleo or "primal" diets have been implemented in order to maintain a healthy weight and GI.[98]

Many healthnuts that go paleo have seen dramatic changes in their health. Some find the diet more energizing. Others see that they are lacking some nutrients that they previously consumed on non-paleo diets, such as grains. However, some studies estimate the original paleo diet consisted of a high level of dietary fiber (100 grams or more). In one study, rats which fed on a fermented fiber in addition to a high-fat paleo diet were found to have reduced appetite and body weight. It is probable that the fiber signals to the brain to suppress appetite.[99] In other words, fiber not only fills you up, but also tells your brain that you're full. This could be one reason why there is improvement in blood sugar response in some studies: fiber slows the indulgence and digestive processes.[100] Paleo also involves a higher percentage of vegetables and animal protein. Although this is great for building lean tissue, it may cause other imbalances by over-consuming proteins.

HEALTHNUT CONS

- Paleo diets may miss some key nutrients by eliminating some healthy foods.
- Paleo diets may decrease fiber consumption with the increases in proteins and fats.
- Paleo diets may encourage higher fat and protein which may lead to other diseases.

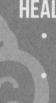

HEALTHNUT PROS

- Paleo encourages whole foods such as healthy fruits, vegetables, seeds, and nuts.
- Paleo proteins and fats may benefit weight and blood sugar balancing.
- Paleo boosts energy through the hunter-gatherer diet and physical activity philosophy.

HEALTHNUT SPECIAL

The three specialty diets are high-plant diets, gluten-free diets, and athletic diets. These diets could also be termed "Popular Diets: Part Two" because of their current trending status! In reality, however, strict adherence to these diets is only for specialized situations or interests. Many dabble, without fully committing, to the beneficial aspects of these diets. Even a vegetarian or vegan might not like everything in the high-plant diet, because it contains some meat. An individual who's not gluten-free may be still interested in some aspects of the gluten-free diet. Similarly, a non-athlete may be interested in some aspects of the athletic diet. Although these three diets do have a themed label, the healthnut can look beyond the label to see what principles can benefit their own individual health plan.

HIGH-PLANT DIETS

High-plant diets are really a combination of mostly plant food combined with some animal and healthy fats. They are great for some healthnuts to control cravings and blood sugar. More specifically, a high-plant diet is a combination of higher protein and higher complex plant carbs with the required amount of fats only taken from healthy sources like avocado or olive oil. Plant diets also build phytonutrient and antioxidant protection in the cells to minimize the progression of the aging process. Furthermore, high-plant diets, along with a small to moderate portion of protein, help to rejuvenate brain cells and add plenty of fiber and healthy fats for optimal nervous system function.

83

PLANT PRIORITY

Tana Amen, wife of popular brain physician Dr. Daniel Amen, describes in her book, *The Omni Diet*, how to make plants the priority of your diet. She advocates consuming non-starch vegetables, small amounts of fruits, and other plant sources of proteins, fats, and carbohydrates. The combination of these plants makes up about 70% of the diet. The other 30% is protein from plants and fish, preferably wild-caught fish. Amen attempts to persuade people off of grains, processed sugar, and other addictive sweeteners.[101]

High-plant diets also take into account the critical microbiota gut and brain connection. It is known that one's diet has a profound impact on gut microbiota. High-plant diets appear to balance appetites and build healthy gut bacteria community. Intestinal permeability is a big problem with our modern SAD diets. It appears we need extra support to close the gaps of the barrage of unhealthy food on our digestive processes and to encourage effective hormonal communication. A diet high in plants and fibrous foods supports intestinal fluidity and feeds beneficial bacteria.[102] The bacterial metabolism and gut hormone signaling is critical to optimize brain function and satiety, signaling when you're full and naturally preventing overindulgence. With the addition of beneficial fats and some animal protein such as fish, there is a greater chance of consuming a wide variety of necessary fat-soluble vitamins and essential minerals.

An example of this diet is found in the diet of the Hadza, an indigenous ethnic group in north-central Tanzania, Africa. The majority of their diet is based on high-fiber plants (70%) and the rest comes from birds and lean, wild game meats. The diet is focused on wild foods such as land vegetables, berries, baobab, honey, and meat. Since this diet is based on the natural whole food habitat, there are no processed meats. Part of the purpose of this diet is to foster an optimal microbiota gut bacteria and, in a sense, it is a version of the hunter-gatherer or paleo dietary profile.[103] However it differs from other hunter-gatherer populations which have a much higher amount of protein and fats and a lower amount of plants. This is the reason I included them as an example of the high-plant category. As you can see, there is such variation even among the dietary themes.

Actually, the high-plant diet at times most closely resembles my personal approach to health—although I freely admit that my diet fluctuates with the different seasons or nutritional requirements throughout the year. Yes, I do modify and adjust in creative dietary fashion. Generally, I try to eat a higher plant-based diet with an adequate amount of protein and healthy fats. There are times when I go on a plant protein and fat whole food binge with nuts and seeds and lower carbs. At other times, however, I'll switch again to balanced ratios of fish, vegetables, and whole grains. Although I do categories, I don't like to stay in categories (must be a healthpreneur thing—or maybe just a human thing!).

If you are a complete vegan and do not include any animal or fish sources of protein, sticking to a strict dietary regimen, you may be lacking in some key nutrients. That's one of the reasons Tana Amen includes adequate protein and healthy fat suggestions in her book, but without overdoing the fats. For example, I've heard her mention that she doesn't usually use oil while cooking unless it is coconut oil. Coconut oil is a medium-chain triglyceride fat that actually helps your body to use fat as energy instead of using it as storage.

HEALTHNUT CONS

- Some high-plant diets may be limited if they don't include enough proteins and fats.
- High-plant diets may not work for some with plant-based digestive difficulties.
- Some high-plant diets may lack key nutrients by eliminating healthy food groups.

HEALTHNUT PROS

- High-plant diets are phytonutrient, chemoprotective, antioxidant, and anti-inflammatory.
- High-plant diets increase beneficial fiber for healthy digestion and waste removal.
- High-plant diets with protein and fats may boost energy, burn fat, and build lean tissue.

GOD DIETS

Another group of high-plant diets are colloquially called "God diets." Most of the God diets are high in plant volume while also containing a combination of clean animal foods. Some God diets are more heavily vegetarian, such as the Hallelujah diet, created by Geòrge Malkmus. This diet eliminates protein and fats from animal sources. Malkmus points to specific scriptural passages, mainly from the Old Testament, to support his theory of vegetarianism.[104] The diet also gets rid of refined foods, hydrogenated oils, refined sugars, caffeine, and alcohol. Furthermore, participants are encouraged to take dehydrated nutritional supplements, such as barley grass juice powder, and to incorporate juicing. In some small scale studies, participants have reported dramatic improvements in their health including reductions in fibromyalgia symptoms, fatigue, and depression.[105] The Hallelujah research associate Michael Donaldson also hypothesizes that this dietary protocol, when combined with specific nutraceuticals is chemoprotective.[106]

However, the proponents of high-plant combined with clean animal sources, such as Jordan Rubin's *New York Times* best seller *The Makers Diet*, point out other scriptural passages that allow for meats, albeit specific types of clean meats.[107] It's incredible how the ancient Hebrews avoided disease with methods not confirmed by the scientific community until centuries later. For example, they prohibited consumption of pork prior to any official discovery of pathogenic parasitic contaminations being officially associated with pigs.[108]

So what is God's diet? Is it vegetarian? Does it not include any shellfish or pork? Is it devoid of raw milk? There are many different opinions and each perspective presents its case studies, reasons, and even research. These opinions must be weighed with what scientific research has unveiled. Much of the scientific literature has established that a high-plant diet, combined with a little animal source protein—without consuming unhealthy animal products—is a balanced approach. Keep in mind the healthnut's foundational principle: the diet you choose should be based on your individual biochemistry, interests, and life season.

Other factors, like emotional and spiritual health, should impact your decision as well. You can eat a clean diet but still have toxic emotions that negatively influence your body, such as anger, frustration, worry, fear, anxiety, or depression. Ask yourself, how might toxic emotions be influencing your health, eating patterns, and nutrient assimilation? At some point, diet is not as important as the health of your mind and emotions.

Although we have much knowledge in terms of physical health, I believe we have only begun to scratch the surface of what is possible from an emotional and spiritual perspective. There is certainly no perfect God diet, other than the principle of eating real foods that God created to be received with thanksgiving.[109] This is not a license for gluttony nor a reason to bless something that God did not create for good! Everything is permissible, but not everything is beneficial.[110] So rest assured that whether vegetarian, omnivore, both, or none—it's your choice!

HEALTHNUT CONS

- God diets may vary in their approach and philosophy depending on their references.
- God diets are often dependent on the beliefs of the one participating in the diet.
- God diets may be somewhat inclusive or restrictive for people.

HEALTHNUT PROS

- God diet views are traditionally higher plant based with moderate or limited animal.
- God diets use scriptural references to support healthier choices.
- God diets may add emotional and spiritual support components, an integral part of true, lasting health.

GLUTEN-FREE DIETS

Gluten is a protein in wheat and other cereal grains, such as barley and rye, that is difficult for some people to digest, acting as an anti-nutrient in the body. Gluten provides the framework for baked products such as bread and other processed foods. However, gluten intolerance and Celiac disease may affect your glands and hormones (such as your thyroid, which is directly involved in your metabolism and energy function). Celiac disease is a small-intestine, autoimmune condition that requires complete elimination of gluten.[111] Although the majority of population has not been confirmed to have Celiac (considered a genetic condition), it is thought that the overabundance of gluten in so many foods other than grain products has had an adverse effect on our society's health and may be causing a gluten intolerance.

The premise behind the wildly popular gluten-free diet is that we generally overconsume grains, especially the wheat that causes food intolerances. According to Dr. William Davis, *New York Times* best-selling author of *Wheat Belly*, Einkorn or Emmer wheat are the only healthy forms of wheat.[112] Unfortunately, these ancient pure grains that are higher in protein have been hybridized and transformed over time into the modern unhealthy gluten wheat we have today. Gluten-free diets may also include corn, rice, gluten-free oats, millet, buckwheat, quinoa, amaranth, and the typical vegetables, fruits, nuts fish, eggs, meats, and other healthy vegetable oils.[113]

For individuals who can digest and assimilate modern wheat and gluten, those foods have been so destroyed by seeds and farming practices that it's not the same grain as it was a long time ago. There are now anti-nutrients that disrupt normal gut balance in your digestive and elimination systems. If your gut is inflamed from gluten or other anti-nutrients, you may experience a negative impact on your brain function and immune system.

MARKETING GLUTEN-FREE

Gluten-free products are flying off the shelves. Unfortunately, many of these products are highly processed and contain other ingredients that are harmful. I was at a health show recently, because I always love finding exciting, new, and healthy products, and I walked by a booth offering specialty desserts. Although the products were labeled gluten-free, these desserts still contained white rice as the main ingredient! As I'll describe in more detail later, white rice is not a nutrient-dense food. I asked the booth tender about it, but she didn't really have much to say other than she was trying to appeal to popular tastes.

Well, food is not about taste first. Taste is second! Most important is nutrition and whether or not the food is digestible and absorbable. Just because a product is gluten-free does not mean it's healthy.

One of the major problems with gluten-free diets is that it is very difficult to avoid traces of gluten. One clinical trial points out that there are major compliance issues in avoiding gluten if you are intolerant or have a condition like Celiac disease.[114] I've discussed with several colleagues how a fraction of gluten particle may cause an inflammatory response in the gut. For example, many restaurants use sauces and spices that contain gluten because it's used as a sifting element. It's extremely difficult to avoid this when eating out and requires long conversations with the server and altogether eliminating certain foods.

Additionally, even products that are naturally gluten-free may be processed on equipment that contains wheat and gluten. Although these manufacturers are supposed to clean the equipment, what guarantee is there that all gluten residue has been removed? That's why manufacturers are designing strictly gluten-free facilities that are guaranteed to be gluten-free. I consulted with another company that was in the process of making this transition because of the market potential for gluten-free foods. They confirmed that even gluten-free labeled food may still contain small amounts of gluten, which is the reason they decided to open a dedicated gluten-free manufacturing facility.

WE'RE ALL GLUTENS

The other major—if not well-received—issue with gluten-free diets is that everyone's not gluten intolerant. I know that's a shocker for those of you that are gluten-free fanatics. Hey, I usually avoid gluten (except when occasionally consuming sprouted versions), but does everyone have a problem with gluten? One small study found that those who consumed a gluten-free diet had less healthy bacteria and more unfriendly bacteria in their gut![115] What if this were a larger study? Would the results be the same? A few questions arise, however, about the reliability of this particular study. Remember that when a food says gluten-free, it may still contain gluten at a very low level. That could have been a factor in this study—the unfriendly bacteria may have been perpetrated by small amounts of gluten.

Some argue that certain gluten-free products are higher glycemic, which may negatively impact blood sugar balance. These gluten-free foods may actually encourage macronutrient caloric consumption of carbohydrates that actually reduce metabolic function, which can be harmful from an OB perspective. Others may just not like the taste of these gluten-free foods![116] As you can see, both sides of the gluten-free diet debate have strong cases.

If you think you are intolerant of gluten, there are advanced tests you can take to determine your level of intolerance. Although some feel these tests are controversial, I know many integrative practitioners that use them successfully with their patients. But you'll have to keep in mind that intolerance levels can change throughout your lifetime.

HEALTHNUT CONS

- Gluten-free is difficult to implement since gluten is hidden in so many foods.
- Gluten-free may not make a difference for some people who are not gluten intolerant.
- Gluten-free may not support a healthy bacterial gut balance (based on limited research).

HEALTHNUT PROS

- Gluten-free is a popular trend with many companies eliminating it from their products.
- Gluten-free diets are effective for those who have some level of gluten intolerance or allergic reaction to gluten.
- Gluten-free clears up symptoms with people who have autoimmune issues.

ATHLETIC DIETS

Athletic diets can be anywhere on a wide spectrum based on the type of sport. Ballerinas are going to eat a much different diet than football players. Even within football, each position requires a different diet. Linemen may consume a lot of food. Wide receivers have to be muscular but also need to be lightning fast. Tennis players require diets for endurance and speed, as do long-distance runners. It's concerning to me that one report in the *Journal of Athletic Training* found approximately 50% of the seventy football players whose blood had been tested had negative results characterized by an unhealthy metabolism![117] This is shocking for those who have barely reached a third or a fourth of their life. Do we need to sacrifice our health for athletic success? Surely there's a balance between athletic achievement and long-term health.

In the past, I've always thought athletic diets required at minimum some form of animal protein whether from egg, fish, or clean land animals. Yet, science is investigating other plant-based forms of athletic diets. There are case study examples of rigorous endurance triathletes who incorporate a raw vegan diet with success. However, critics remark that this only shows the diet may not be disastrous to health and is no better or worse than other diets.[118]

In most cases, an athletic diet demands more nutrients, whether macronutrients or micronutrients, and additional food calories. The simple reason for this requirement is they expend more energy than healthnuts who are not as active.

Another issue that concerns athletes is not eating enough food or the right amount of food. The fact that eating disorders proliferate among athletes is well-documented in the scientific literature. For female athletes, this may lead to a number of issues including menstrual irregularities, osteoporosis, and poor energy levels.[119] Even in men, it is quite clear that diet influences hormone and energy levels regardless of where they are on the athletic diet spectrum.[120] Athletes have other special requirements for recovery and repair in cases of injury. Sometimes athletes need to supplement deficiencies or key areas where they need more nutrition that is not readily available from their food.

When I was an athlete in my younger years (even during power lifting and bodybuilding), I consumed a tremendous amount of food and calories. Although I looked great on the outside, I was toxic at the cellular level. This manifested in different ways over time. I had skin, gut, and energy issues at times. It's taken quite a while to repair the damage done in my late teens and early twenties. Thankfully, much of my physical issues are restored, and I am healthier today than when I was younger.

One special type of athletic diet is bodybuilding. One of my favorite diet and bodybuilding books back when I was bodybuilding in the 1990s was *New York Times* best seller *Body for Life* by Bill Phillips. As a bodybuilding and life coach to me, Bill's company, EAS, and his programs were inspiring for my pursuit of physical health. The pictures, the results, and all of the hype were a motivation to be the best I could physically be.[121] Although I was exposed to the most helpful information I could muster at the time, I made some poor eating choices just because I looked good and thought I was therefore immune from ill-health.

I wasn't considering how the constant influx of calories was overloading my system. Sure, I was surrounded by bodybuilding greats like Bill Pearl who advocated a very strict regimen, but at the time, I didn't really understand his diet discipline. To provide a background, Bill is listed as the best built man of the century. I met Bill while I was working at a fitness facility many years ago. He was somewhat quiet and very unassuming. I recall Bill visiting my work facility numerous times. He was always in the gym early in the morning, at around 5 a.m., and ate a very strict diet. He may have also advocated some periods of fasting.

Unlike Bill, most other bodybuilders I found consumed inordinate amounts of calories and then stripped down with a crash weight diet prior to a show. That kind of diet regimen is very rough on the hormonal and metabolic system over one's lifetime and one of the reasons a bodybuilding or power lifting diet can lead to additional physical ailments with age. Power-lifting diets emphasize consuming a huge amount of calories. Whether bodybuilding or power lifting, the diets are stressful internally no matter what results they produce externally.

The best of these diets involve a very clean, balanced diet. That's probably why Bill Pearl eventually switched to a more lacto-ovo vegetarian diet. He has kept much of his muscle mass even into his advanced years. Bill's eighty-year-old frame and athletic diet counters the belief that you need to consume an inordinate amount of protein from animal sources, although once again, the specifics vary from person to person.

Often we discuss what to consume in terms of optimizing diet for athletes, but in reality it's a balanced lifestyle that leads to optimum performance. Sure, there are elite athletes that may get away without a balanced lifestyle; however, I've seen this catch up with athletes in their later years. The choices we make today will help or harm both short-term performance and long-term lifestyle success.

One vital habit of a balanced lifestyle has little to do with eating: proper rest, recovery, and sleep. Sleep has tremendous benefits, and the lack of quality sleep is inevitably detrimental to performance. Notice I say "quality," because *more* is not always *better*. Sleep is critical for growth, recovery, and repair both physiologically and psychologically. Getting at least six hours per night consistently prevents immune, blood sugar, metabolic, mental, and emotional difficulties and promotes a balanced appetite regulation. In regards to heavy travel or other scheduling that may make it difficult to get adequate rest, even power naps prior to training have positive benefits.[122] In terms of overall diet, one element is certain: elite athletes' diets require a combination of consistent, complete lifestyle disciplines regardless of the choice of diet theme.

HEALTHNUT CONS

- Athletic diets may lead to taking dangerous dietary supplements.
- Athletic diets may be extreme and lead to hormone dysfunction.
- Athletic diets may have higher nutritional requirements.

HEALTHNUT PROS

- Athletic diets that provide clean sources of real food are best.
- Athletic diets create a more active and disciplined lifestyle.
- Athletic diets may help you lower body fat and increase lean muscle.

WHICH DIET?

The purpose of describing several diets is not to say none of them work. They do work, in fact, for different individuals and circumstances. So which diet is right for you? There is no one simple answer—because you are unique! In 2009, *The New England Journal of Medicine* reported the results of reduced calorie diets with varying combinations of fat, proteins, and carbohydrates. After analyzing the 811 overweight adults in this study, researchers found that participants lost weight regardless of the specific diet as long as they reduced energy consumption versus energy they expended.[123] Additional reports indicate that what's even more important than the actual diet type is the adherence to a healthy plan for successful weight management—in other words, the behavioral component: are you going to stick with this?

Dr. David Katz, who is the author of *Disease Proof* and leader of the Yale University Prevention Research Center, compared major diets in an unbiased manner (very difficult to do) to see which was healthiest. He looked at low carb, vegetarian, low-glycemic, Mediterranean, mixed, and paleo. Interestingly, many of these fall within the diet theme categories in this book. His findings? All avoid refined starch, sugars, processed foods, some fats, and are likely to include lean meats, fish, or poultry. The themes promote an increase in plants, focus on eating close to nature, and promote minimally processed foods.[124] In my conversations with Dr. Katz, I concur with his theory about that all themed diets focus on one thing: real food! Pretty simple, huh?

AUTHENTIC DIETING

The science of personalized nutrition through nutrigenomics and personal health dynamics is advancing rapidly. In other words, it's increasingly recognized that people vary in their genetic, microbiome, physiological, and metabolic needs[125]—and I'd add the emotional psychosocial and mind-body needs as well. We have to watch that the cultural pressure to rigidly select a specific diet does not override the fun and spontaneity of continuous diet variety and choice.

Imagine how much more healthy you will be if you consume real food on your real lifestyle plan forever with the freedom to modify and adjust as you go. You'd have a healthy weight and healthy cells at the same time. Here's the thing, if you focus too much on counting calories and tracking those very specific details, you'll end up getting discouraged. That routine becomes monotonous. You won't do it for life. So what you need to do is focus on the behaviors that will organically encourage you to eat the right foods and participate in the right physical activities that you enjoy and love.

This is what the Healthnut Life is all about! You create the plan that works for you, as long as you utilize more energy than you consume. (You don't have to count calories—but if you for some reason love tracking those numbers, by all means, do it!) It's that simple. This is exactly how healthnuts maintain their personalized healthy body fat and weight for life: They continually consume less or use more energy than they consume, but they do it without thinking about it!

Although this book does not cover exercise and energy expenditure, healthnuts have a simple choice of regularly participating in the physical activity they are most interested in. Why? Studies suggest the activity you love is the activity you'll do forever. I love what Dr. Michael Roizen, Chief Wellness Officer of Cleveland Clinic and award-winning author of *This Is Your Do-Over*, offers just about the simplest exercise ever: walk 10,000 steps each day.[126] It's one of the easiest exercises to address OB! If you can't do any other exercise—you can at least walk! Maybe even get a treadmill desk! Better yet, do it with a partner (we'll get to that later in the book).

If you start an exercise program for the short term, you'll get bored. However, if you decide to incorporate activities that you love, such as swimming or walking, on a regular basis, it's highly probable you'll naturally achieve the right weight and body fat levels you were designed for. You can have incredible results by doing all of this, including eating like a healthnut—that is, eating real food. As Harvard scientists Drs. Willett and Hu pithily point out in an article about diet reports and the summation of nutrition research over thirty years, "The choice is yours."[127]

HEALTHNUTS...

- Understand a wide variety of diets work to reduce risks of disease and OB.
- Do the personalized lifestyle plan that provides freedom from OB for life.
- Participate in physical activity which complements a healthy diet.

WANT TO KNOW MORE ABOUT ANY OF THESE DIETS?
JOIN THE HEALTHNUT COMMUNITY BY VISITING **DRHEALTHNUT.COM**
TO INQUIRE ABOUT YOUR FAVORITE DIET THEMES.

SCAN TO VISIT DRHEALTHNUT.COM

PART THREE:

DR. HEALTHNUT NO-NO'S

7

HEALTHNUT TOXINS

Toxic food is like that frightening little insect, the wood tick. Slowly and silently, it attaches itself to your life, and quietly sucks the life out of you. You don't even notice it's there—until it might be too late! Toxic food seeps its poison into your cells, tissues, organs, and body slowly, over years. Toxic food is any food that has been refined, processed, chemically altered, or transformed, including genetically modified "Frankenfood," fake food, or anything that is not genuine God-made food.

UNDERSTANDING TOXINS

Before we can understand why it's important to avoid toxic food, we first need a basic understanding of toxins and what they do to us. All humans have an intestinal mucosal barrier that functions like a second skin. Extending from mouth to anus, the barrier is the first line of defense against pathogens and signals when an immune response is needed. More positively, it also allows assimilation of food and nutrients. A healthy intestinal barrier is essential for optimal immune function, for healthy gut function, and for proper digestion and absorption of food. Toxins mess with the intestinal barrier, and therefore mess up your immune system, your gut, and your digestion and absorption of food.

Bacterial toxins in particular can stimulate the immune system to set off a low-grade inflammation, which inhibits or even prevents the barrier from doing its job. Toxic food can make the barrier more permeable, allowing "unscreened" substances into the bloodstream. Heavy metal toxicity, or exposure to heavy metals such as mercury or lead, tears down the barrier and shuts down healthy gut function because the body reacts so strongly to it. The intestinal barrier is able to handle toxins—indeed, it is *designed* to handle toxins! However, when wave after wave of a variety toxins attack the intestinal barrier, the intestinal barrier falls, succumbing the body to disease and dysregulation. It's always the symphony of toxic stresses that is most destructive.[128]

And there's no way around it: we live in a toxic generation. Living a healthy lifestyle and eating properly is more challenging in this century than ever before. We live longer but seem to be unhealthier than any generation before us. The contributors to these toxins are both in and out of our control and may include your occupation, whether or not you smoke, use illicit drugs, or alcohol, relational aspects, social and community factors, environmental exposure to UV rays, or other psychosocial factors such as depression and anxiety.[129]

TOXIC PAIR: ENDOGENOUS OR EXOGENOUS

There are two types of environmental toxins associated with OB: endogenous toxins and exogenous toxins. Endogenous toxins are located inside your body. Exogenous toxins are found outside of your body—including your home and your outside environment.

One of the largest contributors to the OB epidemic and reduced quality of life are environmental toxins—exogenous toxins. With the rapid growth of technology, manufacturing, and energy products in the twentieth century came an abundance of toxins that promote mercury, lead, and arsenic accumulation in humans. These three lethal substances alone are some of the most toxic elements on the planet, according to the CDC environmental health sciences division.[130] Highly specialized lab testing indicates that higher than normal levels of these toxic elements are found in this generation's tissues. Dr. Garry Gordon, an authority and pioneer of integrative medicine, emphasizes that lead is a huge problem today, although mainstream media has downplayed the threat.[131] Dr. Gordon agrees with evidence of toxic element accumulation in a recent Harvard study linking bone lead to higher risks of cardiovascular disease.[132]

Hopefully, once you are on a healthy eating plan, your body can better process and eliminate the external, or exogenous, toxins. However, there really is no safe level of exogenous toxins. These toxins are just a part of our world. We limit them as much as possible, but because external toxins are beyond our control, we must focus our efforts on endogenous toxins, the toxins that we *choose* to consume.

Your body attempts to eliminate endogenous toxins from any fat stores. If you're struggling with OB, these toxins are likely stored in your fat cells. One popular example of endogenous toxins that you may be familiar with is sugar—in the form of dietary fructose. This compound has been linked to OB and other strange metabolic conditions.[133] The goal is to alleviate this pernicious accumulation by reducing or eliminating these toxins so your body can properly assimilate good nutrition and dispose of the wastes effectively. The means to this goal is by limiting the amount of toxic exposure. As the saying goes, "Prevention is better than cure." If you stop consuming toxic food now, you'll lower the chance of OB and other lifestyle diseases during your lifetime.

But how do you know the difference between real food and toxic food? I base my definition of *toxic* on the substance's likelihood of causing harm. For example, if you consume a huge amount of water, it may cause seizures or even death. But is that likely? Of course not! So water is not toxic—rather, it's vital. Even something good for us could become quite toxic if we take it in large doses. Toxic food is not just the wrong food, but food in the wrong amount.

EWG ANALYSIS

You may wonder what proof I have that these endogenous and exogenous toxins could possibly make OB worse. Well, the reason we know toxicity is prevalent in society and has the potential to greatly influence OB is because we have access to a study that shows the effect of endogenous toxins on bodies that are as yet untouched by exogenous toxins. The study documents the toxin accumulation in ten fetuses—who had no exposure to the outside world.

The Environmental Working Group's (EWG) study analyzed the blood of ten embryos to determine how much toxicity was present in their little developing bodies. The results were astounding. Over two hundred toxins were discovered during analysis of the blood samples.[134] The only real toxin source was the toxins coming from the mothers. How did the mothers get these toxins? They received them from internal and external sources. The sad part is that the toxins were not only endogenous but exogenous. The toxins were so concentrated, they infiltrated the fetus tissues inside the womb. If those ten fetuses, never exposed to the outside environment, contain toxins from the mother's blood, what levels are you and I (in our modern era of daily exposure to pollutants and chemicals) open to?

Although this book is not meant to be the ultimate guide to toxicity, it is important to address this topic as it relates to OB. The better your body efficiency in processing and eliminating toxicity, the better chance you have at living a healthy lifestyle free of OB.

HEALTHNUTS...

- Test for heavy metal toxicity with the appropriate measures.
- Eliminate or reduce toxins for effective weight and body fat management.
- Reduce exposure to endogenous and exogenous toxins (as much as you can control).

HEALTHNUT MANIPULATION

I hope it is clear that although toxic food is prevalent, healthnuts must avoid it at all costs. One of the most destructive forms of toxic food is found in man-made genetically modified food (GM food). You may or may not have heard of the term GMO, which stands for "genetically modified organisms." According to the World Health Organization, GMOs (through the technology of "genetic engineering," "gene technology," or "modern biotechnology") are "organisms in which the genetic material (DNA) has been altered in a way that does not occur naturally by mating and/or natural recombination."[135] The purpose is to make the plants more resistant to diseases or pests or more tolerant of herbicides like glyphosate. The result is genetically modified crops, or GM food.

TOXIN CONTRIBUTOR #1: GENETICALLY MODIFIED FOOD

To explain it simply, scientists had the idea of making food better by genetically manipulating seeds and transferring, mixing, or distributing unrelated species. Despite the noble ambition to feed the world with higher quality seeds, plants, and ultimately food, scientists are discovering major problems with this approach. The danger associated with foods grown through genetically modified seeds are significant.[136]

A recent report titled "GMO Myths and Truths" provides an evidence-based examination of the faulty health claims of GMOs, GM foods, and GM crops.[137] In the report the authors discuss the following:

- GM crops are treated with chemicals such as glyphosate.

- GMOs are not bred naturally.

- GM crops decrease nutritional and nutrient quality.

- GM foods are not rigorously tested with multinational, long-term studies.

- GM foods are toxic and not safe to eat.

- GMO regulations are nominal.

- GM food companies restrict availability and access to products by independent researchers.

- GM crops decrease soil quality.

- GM foods increase malnutrition and poverty.

- GMOs cause lowered crop yields.

- GM foods are more expensive to produce than non-GMO natural breeding.

- GM crops contaminate organic and non-GMO crops.

- GM farming accounts for only 12% of available land and less than 1% of all farming.

- GM seeds reduce choices for farmers in the US, Brazil, and India.

- GM crops increase the need for more pesticides, herbicides, and insecticides.

- GMOs damage key organisms and biodiversity while requiring more energy.

- GM foods spike health care costs and will increase disease risks globally.

- GM food is not required to be labeled as such in the US.

- GM foods do not meet the FDA's GRAS (generally regarded as safe) level.

- GM crops disrupt local sustainable and biodynamic agriculture.

NOT YOUR GRANDMOTHER'S POPCORN

Things have certainly changed since I grew up. Gone are the days of going to movies and buying popcorn and feeling good about it. Sure, the popcorn when I was a kid was loaded with a ton of butter and salt, but at least the corn was real back then! Today, it's genetically altered just like many of the popular, commercially processed crops such as sugar beets (a main source of sugar), soybeans, corn, cotton, papaya, and canola.[138] Consider canola as one example. Much of the alteration of canola oil's composition is designed to delay the ripening of the canola plant and resist virus and bacteria—which sounds great, until you realize that the result is worse for our bodies than the original problem.

Genetic modification will not stop with these foods. The popular, commercially processed crops find their way into the ingredient list of hundreds of products. According to the Non-GMO Project, some examples include amino acids, aspartame, ascorbic acid, sodium ascorbate, vitamin C, citric acid, sodium citrate, ethanol, flavorings (both natural and artificial), high-fructose corn syrup, hydrolyzed vegetable protein, lactic acid, maltodextrins, molasses, monosodium glutamate (MSG), sucrose, textured vegetable protein (TVP), xanthan gum, vitamins, and yeast products.[139]

And although grains are not traditionally GMO, they too have been genetically altered.[140] Even grains that supposedly don't have the high levels of gluten end up causing reactions in some gluten sensitive individuals. It's no coincidence that so many inflammatory and autoimmune conditions have sprung up in our population over the last twenty years! Moreover, we've seen a surge in the OB crisis within the same timeframe. Is there a connection? I believe the GMOs and the genetically spliced foods are significant contributors to the OB conundrum.

GLYPHOSATE LYNCH

However, GMOs are not alone in their global threat to healthy eating. Glyphosate, a broad spectrum toxic herbicide used to control or manipulate undesirable plants and the evil twin to genetically modified food, can be found in many well-known brands. Glyphosate products are advertised as being safe, but this could not be further from the truth. A recent experiment with aquatic life found that glyphosate is understated in its toxicity effects on reproductive viability in these invertebrate life forms. How much more destructive could it be for human reproductive capabilities?[141]

The prestigious medical journal *The Lancet Oncology* reported that the World Health Organization (WHO) found that the herbicide glyphosate "probably" causes cancer in humans. The chemical has been found in the blood and urine of agricultural workers as it spreads through spraying, water, and food.[142] Glyphosate and other complementary chemicals are neurotoxic and induce cancer cells through estrogenic activity.[143] These chemicals do not support life. They only destroy it.

The glyphosate story hit home for me a number of years ago. We lived in a community that endeavored to start a local garden. *What an exceptional idea!* I thought. I am a big proponent of growing and purchasing local foods to the max. However, when I found out the garden would allow the use of glyphosate and other pesticides and herbicides, I called the director to inquire the reason. I specifically asked why they would take such a great idea and subvert it with this chemical. He responded, "There is no problem with glyphosate. It only stays in the soil for a limited time and then it vanishes." Vanishes? It just disintegrates in the ground? I could not believe what I was hearing.

I then went to a local organic and biodynamic farmer and asked him the same question. He just looked at me and shook his head at the glyphosate predicament. "No, it's not going away," he said.

The research supports this farmer's statement. In one of the most thorough studies to date on GM toxicity, rats consumed GM foods along with glyphosate. The conclusion? Rats that ate the genetically modified food with pesticides had kidney, hormonal, and liver failure along with a plethora of tumors.[144] After going through an independent peer review and confirmed by scientists globally, the study was retracted from the journal editor based on peer pressure from lobbyists and other paid proponents of GM food. Yet the fact remains, the results were statistically significant regarding organ damage and hormonal disruption in these rats, and these results were never thoroughly disputed by the study's retractors.

GLYPHOSATE EVIDENCE FROM "GMO MYTHS AND TRUTHS"

The data is growing. The same analysis I mentioned before from "GMO Myths and Truths" also reported on an herbicide product that uses glyphosate as an active ingredient (along with the insecticide endotoxin Bt used to kill pests from the inside out):[145]

- Glyphosate-based products cause increased health risks that can lead to birth defects.

- Glyphosate causes cellular toxicity.

- Glyphosate product studies are antiquated and biased in their funding.

- Glyphosate products confuse normal plant function and kill soil organisms.

- Bt found in GM crops is toxic to human cells and disrupts the immune, reproductive, and digestive systems.

- Bt shows toxicity in multiple other organ systems and also contributes to OB.

Additionally, a recent report from the Netherlands describes an adverse decision against a well-known glyphosate-based herbicide product because of misinformation regarding its safety. The report details the decision and documents how the company that produces the product did not respond to the adverse claims.[146] In effect, the committee states that the company that manufactures the herbicide product is pleading guilty.[147] To provide further documentation of this decision, a report published in *Entropy* confirms that the infestation of glyphosate contributes to preventable diseases.

The authors suggest glyphosate may be the most toxic and "biologically disruptive chemical in our environment." Furthermore glyphosate disrupts the cytochrome P450 enzyme that shuts down detoxification pathways creating additional toxicity through the body. In effect, the authors suggest that glyphosate causes or worsens "gastrointestinal disorders, obesity, diabetes, heart disease, depression, autism, infertility, cancer" and Alzheimer's.[148] Glyphosate is likely linked to every modern, degenerative, chronic lifestyle disease known to mankind and is probably the most biologically disruptive chemical in the history of humanity!

HEALTHNUTS...

- Avoid crops with chemicals like the insecticide Bt.
- Avoid glyphosate-based products and their derivatives.
- Avoid GMOs and support the non-GMO movement.

THE DISASTER OF THE TWENTY-FIRST CENTURY

Within the last twenty years, GMOs have been a tragic example of profit potential at the expense of humans, animals, and the environment. GMOs are on a mission, knowingly or unknowingly, to destroy population. That includes you! Does it really matter whether the companies promoting GMOs truly know the danger of their products? If they do, you are in trouble. If they don't, you are in trouble. Either way, it's going to be a problem for you, unless you take responsibility for your health and rise up as a voice for clean food.

How did we allow GMOs to permeate our world? The GMO approach is really no different in kind than the approach of the pharmaceutical industry. People take pills to alleviate mental stress or pain. The pill doesn't provide a cure; it just temporarily stops the symptoms. It does not get to the root cause and may cause additional symptoms. The same is true with GMO seeds. The seeds become "drugged up." Where do the drugs go? Into your body. What effect do they have on your organs, your systems, and your lifestyle? It's not yet fully documented, and yet despite concerns, most of us consume them wholesale. However, where pharmaceuticals can be very beneficial for a period of time in a crisis, emergency, or non-lifestyle based chronic disease situation, GM foods are never a solution for any situation.

Think about the effects of pharmaceuticals on the body. Nutrient depletions occur with every drug that you take. Dr. Ross Pelton, an internationally known integrative pharmacist, describes this nutrient depletion phenomenon in his exhaustive work, *The Drug Induced Nutrient Depletion Handbook*. In addition to the side effects from taking drugs, Pelton specifies the exact nutrients that will be depleted. Compound this depletion with multiple prescriptions, and the body becomes severely malnourished.[149] Why would this nutrient depletion with pharmaceuticals not be similar to artificially engineered or genetically obstructed GMOs? Could this massive science experiment disrupt the health of many in exchange for the profit of a few?

UN-LABELED

Even if you are convinced to try to buy fewer GM products, how do you know if the food you are eating contains GMOs? The Grocery Manufacturers Association estimates up to 70%–80% of the foods consumed in the US contain GMs.[150] Many of these foods likely contain GM corn, soybeans, or sugar beets found in packaged or processed foods and are not healthy.

Unfortunately, most stores don't adopt GM labeling, which begins with the number eight on a produce label sticker. That question is further complicated by the fact that some parties have a vested interest in keeping you from being informed. During the November 2012 election, California instituted a ballot for mandatory labeling of GMOs on every food (Proposition 37). What was the result? The bill was rejected, thanks to the marketing and advertising efforts of companies in favor of GMO use.[151]

The trend continued in another vote in 2013 when the majority of senators voted against amending the farm bill to require GMO labeling. Was there anything extraordinary in the requiring GMOs to be labeled? Senator Bernie Sanders (I-VT) described the amendment request to label GMOs as "fairly common sense," considering that the EU and other countries all over the world support consumer food awareness measures.[152]

More recently, the bill H.R. 1599, or the Safe and Accurate Food Labeling Act of 2015, has been proposed. Although the proposal may seem to bring more labeling transparency, it does not. The bill seeks to ban states from requiring companies to comply with the mandatory labeling of GMOs. States such as Maine, Connecticut, and Vermont have already passed laws that require GM foods to be labeled. There are twenty-six states that are considering GMO labeling laws, which is why it is critical other states come on board. Perhaps this national bill is being fronted now to prevent any other states from passing labeling laws. However, celebrities, business leaders, and advocates are championing mandatory GM labeling in spite of this bill.

Are the people and legislators who voted in each of these measures truly educated about the dangers of GMOs? Or did they just vote because of some benefit or their pocketbook? We may never know, but what we do know is that there is more of an uprising every day among the rest of us who want to know what's in our food and to have the ability to choose it without undue complication. As Representative Jim McGovern (D-MA) said in an article from USA TODAY, "people ought to get what they want, to know what is in their food."[153] He goes on to question why these GM industry proponents are pushing so hard to prevent mandatory labeling. It's like they have something to hide!

Thankfully, some big companies are stepping up to the plate for the public good. Whole Foods is mandating labeling of GMO foods for their stores within the next several years (to be completed by 2018).[154] No matter what you think about Whole Foods or any other company that has both healthy and less healthy products and services in their stores, their decision to properly label their foods is a huge step in the right direction. I applaud their leadership on this particular matter.

Others, like Trader Joe's and Chipotle, are offering non-GMO products as well. Regardless of what each state decides about GMO labeling regulations, I expect to see other stores and restaurants will follow the non-GMO trend during the next twenty years. I predict grocery stores, markets, eateries, restaurants, and packaged foods will comply regardless of regulation and simply because of public demand. The massive public uprising will be so great that people will demand to know what is, or is not, in their foods.

Although there are no GM animals approved for human consumption yet, a genetically modified salmon is currently being proposed to the FDA. It will likely to be approved soon. Other major companies are standing up to the GM lobby. The two largest grocery stores in the US, Safeway and Kroger, will not sell GM salmon. The pressure is now on large warehouses like Costco to not give in to the GM threats as there are numerous other genetically engineered fish being "manufactured" globally.[155]

HEALTHNUTS...

- Observe the environment and facts surrounding GMO claims.
- Understand GMOs can act like drugs with side effects on the body.
- Push for foods to be labeled properly and know that *more* food doesn't mean *better* food.

WHAT IF?

Remember, *you* have the power! *You* are the government in this land and control what occurs in terms of laws and statutes. No matter where you live, you should have the right to know what's in your food and where it came from. Can you imagine a nation full of healthnuts purchasing only non-GMO food? Can you imagine if there were labeling requirements for GMO foods for every grocery store, every restaurant, and every dispensary of food? Only the producers of quality would survive and thrive. This is real economics; this is the principle of supply and demand for the best products at work. This type of capitalism, the capitalism that produces a healthier population with healthier healthnuts, is what I'm all for. I'm not for capitalism that harms the environment or population or causes destruction.

As you can probably infer, I support at least labeling, perhaps restricting, and maybe even all-out banning genetically modified or engineered foods. The large-scale food industry is corrupted. GMO advertising is pervasive. Those colorful boxes of kid's cereals, that even adults love to consume, are produced with cheap modified ingredients. Marketers make money off of ignorance. Health-care insurers and organizations make money off of the same ignorance. They don't expect you to find out the truth.

However, although advertisers control what is marketed, we are in charge of the food demand. You can choose to eat the right foods regardless of your economic state. Ultimately, you have a right to know the most critical information about that food you consume on a regular basis so you can make the most informed choice.

Remember the garden my community tried to start? I had a right to know what chemicals were used. Guess what? It didn't really matter that they thought they could take a shortcut by using chemicals. Here's how that story ended—the garden no longer exists today! Once again, this demonstrates how the marketing and advertising of misinformation influences the gatekeepers of health in our society.

We need to change that. You are now the gatekeeper of health and a part of this healthnut movement that our nation, our cities, and our communities so desperately need. The information is not limited to the few but to the masses. Remember, being a healthnut is not about being crazy; it's just about being passionate about being healthy so you and your loved ones may live with vitality. Therefore, you have a responsibility, as I'm charging you, a healthnut, to go and make a difference in your communities and organizations.

HEALTHNUTS...

- Skip the snacks that are GM or genetically engineered.
- Are seldom fooled by deceptive marketing gimmicks.
- "Vote" for real food and real health by their purchases.

9

HEALTHNUT FAKES

The second most destructive contributor to toxicity is processed foods. We are now seeing a shift to convenience foods that align with a fast-paced lifestyle in both developed countries and developing nations.[156] Processed and refined foods have inundated just about every sphere of global society over the past thirty years, and are defined as foods that have been milled, grinded, or processed in some form.

TOXIN CONTRIBUTOR #2: PROCESSED AND REFINED FOODS

Whole foods, because they are bioactive, are recommended over refined foods.[157] These bioactive parts of the foods are like all of the parts of your car. Without them, you are missing something important and your car won't work properly. When everything is tuned up right, the car works great. Refined foods are like cars stripped of all their essential parts—no fuel tank, no tail pipe, no engine. Similarly, refined foods strip all the essential components that your body knows how to process. With only refined foods, your body has no fuel, no way to burn the fuel, and no ability to move forward.

Refined foods include sugar-engorged waters, fruit drinks, carbonated beverages, and other liquid delights. Refined foods may include frozen potato products, ready-to-eat cereals, and frozen on-the-go foods, and are usually found in stores in lower to middle income areas. These venues rarely offer any significant whole food, vegetable, or fruit choices. Instead, they offer processed, high-fat, sodium, and added-sugar foods.[158] That's what I consumed my during my teen years! I didn't know, then, what I was doing to my body. Refined foods are a segment of processed foods that can be very unhealthy.

We've seen this principle demonstrated in studies comparing whole grains to refined grains. Refined carbohydrates such as white rice and wheat products have been associated with an increased risk of cardiovascular disease independent of other societal risk factors because they promote a faster rise in blood glucose. The body doesn't have to break it down. This is another reason why OB, low-grade inflammation, and diabetes often go hand in hand.[159] Clearly, the whole grain reduces bad fat while the refined grain increases bad fat and high levels of undesirable LDL particle carriers of cholesterol.[160] Regardless what you believe about gluten in whole grains, the evidence is clear that real food has the potential to impact weight and even blood lipid levels.

WHOLE FOODS VERSUS STRIPPED FOODS

Diets that consistently include refined foods are linked to obesity and cardiovascular disease.[161] There is a caveat to the food refining process, however. If you take a whole grain, such as millet for example, and cook the millet in its raw form, it's unlikely to cause a major spike in blood sugar. The millet will also contain the fiber beneficial for slowing your digestion. If you take that same millet and you grind it up into a fine powder, it is still nutritious to a degree, but will probably load faster into your bloodstream because your digestion and absorption rates will increase. The millet has already been broken down and your body didn't have to do as much work.

Millet, however, still contains a high nutritional value and is not as unhealthy as a doubly or triply refined product, such as white rice flour. Let me explain. With white rice, you are starting with an anti-nutrient. So if you further refine the white rice, it doesn't get healthier, but rather unhealthier. White rice is missing various nutritional constituents because it's not a whole grain, like brown rice is. White rice is stripped of vital phytonutrients and fiber in the bran and outer germ layers and is "polished" to leave only the starchy endosperm with losses in protein, fat, vitamins, and other antioxidant activity.[162] The result is a nutrient-devoid food. In cohort studies of thousands of US men and women, brown rice is associated with a small risk for type 2 diabetes while white rice was a larger risk for type 2 diabetes.[163] To some degree, whole foods versus stripped foods follow this same pattern that is seen in millet versus white rice and white rice flour.

The pattern can also be seen in other foods. If you believe all fats are equal, for example, then you would certainly stay away from nuts, which are high in fats. However, more recent evidence reveals that consuming nuts can actually have beneficial effects on weight and triglyceride levels.[164] Some say cholesterol levels are the vital factor in determining an individual's unhealthy fat level. However, it is triglycerides, or blood fat levels, that are really the most important factor in determining the state of your health. You can have higher total cholesterol and low triglycerides and be healthier than someone who has lower total cholesterol but higher triglyceride levels.

This is because triglycerides are the actual fats in your blood. A refined carbohydrate-containing nutrient may actually increase your body's fat storage capacity compared to a food that is mostly fat. That's why you can consume pistachios—a mostly fat food that's low in triglycerides—versus a refined, carbohydrate-containing pretzel, and still be slender and at a healthy weight. Isn't that amazing?

Don't get me wrong! I'm not saying to overindulge on the nuts! I am saying that you can eat a controlled amount of nuts and feel full without the side effects of the refined processed foods that lead to more hunger and indulging food addictions.

HEALTHNUTS...

- Avoid bad carb foods that are stripped of nutrients.
- Snack on healthy whole or real food "snacks."
- Stick to low GI and low GL foods for blood sugar balance.

Processing strips the food of nutrients and is a leading cause of underlying digestive inflammation. Most of the corn, wheat, soy, and dairy have been processed into oblivion because food and nutrition scientists were intending to create tasty, affordable, and good food.[165] But these processed foods actually become toxic missiles to your immune system. Refined grains contribute to insulin resistance and destroy blood sugar balance. Your body cannot handle such a rush of glucose, not kept in check by insulin that after having been "fired upon" is now defunct. Couple this with an inactive or slow lifestyle and you have a double dose of disaster.

THE NEMESIS OF YOUR GUT

Dr. Mark Hyman, author of *New York Times* best seller *The Blood Sugar Solution*, directly addresses the millions of diagnosed and undiagnosed diabetics by describing the cause and solution to protect against diabetes. In his best seller, he claims that highly processed foods, such as wheat, contain the protein gluten—which has a different chemical makeup than the gluten in yesteryear's bread, as we've mentioned before. The sticky gluten protein invades one's digestive tracts,[166] and the immune system may react inappropriately. Sometimes, hole-like gaps form in one's intestines after eating too many processed foods. This is often termed as "leaky gut." The easiest solution is to remove these offending foods from the patient's diet.

If you think you may be suffering from leaky gut, it's best to test your food intolerance levels. Whether it is gluten or another processed food causing low-grade inflammation, remove it from your diet!

For example, I used to eat a significant amount of processed protein shakes when I was younger. I would consume tubs and tubs of denatured whey protein to build lean muscle tissue. However, I was completely ignoring the harmful effects this perpetuated on my gut. The overconsumption of a specific food became a problem. The protein no longer was a friend, but an invisible enemy. The little proteins became like invaders in my body, causing gas, bloating, and other disturbances in my mid-section. It wasn't until I completely removed the whey protein from my diet that the distressing symptoms began to dissipate. Eliminating these products was a difficult decision. I liked having my protein smoothies every morning, and the cravings were nearly unbearable.

You may have experienced this feeling with your favorite foods as well. Although I knew from my studies and work with practitioners that it's important to rotate foods, there was a gap in my life between knowing and doing. I needed to incorporate the healthnut *Aha!* into my lifestyle. See, I've always had the power to choose what I want to consume or not. I just don't always make the smart choice. The same is true for you. You have the same power every day to make the right choices for your lifestyle. The good news is that one mistake—or even a dozen mistakes!—cannot disqualify you for life. Tomorrow always contains a new chance. But if a lifetime of tomorrows go by with no change, those little repeated mistakes will destroy your body.

HEALTHNUTS...

- Avoid processed foods in order to build digestive efficiency.
- Avoid processed foods for optimal nutrient absorption.
- Avoid processed foods for proper immune system function.

HEALTHY PROCESSED FOODS?

Dr. Robert Lustig in his *New York Times* best seller *Fat Chance* depicts processed foods as the main culprit in OB. Surprised? *You* might not be the primary culprit in the equation.[167] People do not choose to be OB. They are bombarded with marketing for unhealthy and toxic food, and they don't know the difference. To a large extent, I would agree with Dr. Lustig's claims about unhealthy processed foods—especially when considering recent research that the artificial ingredient of sugar. OB is not necessarily as simple as energy intake of calories and energy expenditure of calories. Another complexity is that processed food adds sugar as just one more artificial ingredient. The problem's been understated because unnatural sweeteners and sugar, like other processed foods, are highly addictive and toxic.[168]

However, here I must digress and give credence to a small percentage of processed foods that are in fact healthy. What? Am I contradicting myself? No, it's really true, some foods are healthily processed. A banana blended with water, spinach, ground chia seeds, ice, and some berries is processed but not necessarily unhealthy. Why? Because it's processed with real food, not toxic food. If you take a whole food and process it in a high-powered blender, you are simply making it more palatable. The nutrition is still there. Even if a food is juiced, it can still be processed healthily. The fiber may be removed through the juice processing, but the real nutritional benefits will absorb more readily into your bloodstream. That doesn't mean you should juice 10,000 carrots and drink it in one sitting! There is a balanced approach to everything. Likewise, consuming a large amount of fruit and especially freshly juiced fruit over an extended period of time is probably not a good idea for blood sugar balance. My point is that it's possible to process things healthily oneself.

However, the natural sugar found in whole fruits with fiber is not the same as eating a donut that is highly processed toxic food. The same is true for the highly processed white rice transformed into white flour as mentioned earlier. These ultra-processed foods are considered unhealthy, and are very different from throwing a banana with fiber in the blender.[169] The next level of processed foods is typically fast foods and those are advertised as quick fixes. Make no mistake about it. Advertising and promotion of fast food restaurants play a large role in luring people into consuming these unhealthy processed foods regularly.[170] The mass, continual broadcasting of these marketing messages contributes to the OB epidemic. Just remember, a processed food that is a toxic food is in its own unhealthy category.

HEALTHNUTS...

- Only process whole real foods for nutritional benefit.
- Keep fiber intact when processing foods.
- Avoid unhealthy, processed, refined foods or fake foods.

PACKAGED FOODS

Processed foods are often found in packages, and such packaged foods seem to have taken over supermarkets. Why are the inner aisles of grocery stores the most food-packed yet least nutritionally dense? The inner aisles also make up the majority of the shopping experience at most stores. A new report from *BMJ* describes the link between packaged foods and OB.[171]

The truth is that food preservation has taken over our food culture. It's easy to buy food that is easily stored and to store food that is easily purchased. Granted, there is a time and place for easily stored food. Sometimes, convenience is important, too. But the decision to go with packaged products should not be the norm in your regular food consumption. Your goal should be to consume as much fresh or frozen food as possible.

Some claim that convenience foods make it easier to track portions—I only ate one bar, or one box—with the result that one consumes less. However, the problem lies not in the *quantity* but the *quality* of that packaged food. Is it sustainable to eat small portions of unhealthy food over a long period of time—over your whole life?

The other problem with claiming that convenience food's packaging limits intake is that, according to a *New York Times* article on the science of junk food, it's well known by savvy marketers that packaged salty, sugary, and fatty foods are addictive to taste buds and the brain.[172] Chances are that you won't stop at one bar, or one box. Ultimately, if you buy junk foods, you set your brain up for the frying pan.

PACKAGED DENSITY

The healthiest, most nutrient-dense foods on the planet are fresh or frozen. Contrast that with a preserved food that is highly likely to contain artificial, synthetic, or chemically altered foods. It is well-known within the food industry that food packaging, such as plastics, contain harmful chemicals that inevitably enter the food to some extent.[173] This is consistent with the rise of Bisphenol-A or BPA toxicity awareness. Examples of packaged foods that are beneficial are those that dehydrate real foods under 115 degrees and are able to confirm their nutritional statements on their label and food preparation practices. If a food is preserved below this temperature, then it's likely that a good percentage of the vital nutritional enzymes and phytochemicals are intact. The enzymes are what make the food not only digestible but also absorbable and utilizable in your body. If you can't use the nutrients, there's no point to eating them!

That's why some people have to take digestive enzymes all the time. They've displaced their pancreatic enzyme functionality and other digestive organs from properly producing and utilizing digestive enzymes. If we focus on eating nutrient-dense, enzymatic-rich foods, we're at a lower risk for needing to consume digestive enzymes (although certain health conditions may still require them).

Inevitably, eating the wrong kinds of packaged foods will deplete enzymes on a macro level because of the disruption to the digestive, endocrine, and neurological systems. Eating the right types of packaged foods will contribute to proper nutrient assimilation, hormonal balance, and healthy brain function. Typically, these healthy packaged foods are found at specialty or natural food stores, depending on where you live. There are some mainstream grocers that are starting to carry more of these healthier options as well. Of course, you can make your own, but that is laborious if your schedule is already packed.

Most importantly, in terms of packaged foods, it is critical to understand that a knowledge of food labels alone will not change your behavior.[174] Behavioral change involves a focused determination and action plan that is practically lived out day by day with accountability from like-minded individuals.

HEALTHNUTS...

- Avoid unhealthy packaged foods that contain processed ingredients.
- Buy healthy packaged foods that are whole and have to be refrigerated or frozen.
- Eat healthy, dried packaged goods that are preservative-free.

HEALTHNUT IMITATORS

The third most destructive contributor to toxicity is conventional food, which is usually made with ingredients that contain synthetic fertilizers, biocides, growth regulators, and, through livestock feed, antibiotics, growth hormones, and other additives that are not meant for human consumption. This leads to higher amounts of pesticide residues and heavy metal contamination in these conventional foods. There are links between pesticide exposure and health risks like cancer, neurological problems, and reproductive issues.[175]

Does organic food contain more nutrients than conventionally grown food? Well, there is not yet enough evidence to decide either way. However, what's far more critical is the likelihood, not that conventional food has fewer nutrients, but that it has far more chemicals; and the interactions of these nutrients and toxins in the body can have lasting negative effects.[176]

TOXIN CONTRIBUTOR #3: CONVENTIONAL FOODS

Conventional food is a term used for the unhealthy way food is normally grown, as opposed to the way food should be grown. Of course, I have high hopes that soon organically grown will be the "conventional" way. Until then, however, healthnuts need to speak out and live out a healthier way. Although specific human investigations of conventional versus organic are not plentiful, does it take fifty studies and a multi-year meta-analysis to demonstrate that conventionally grown food may harm us? I don't want to wait that long to find out, and I think most healthnuts don't want to, either. Some researchers try to say that conventionally grown food is just as healthy or nutritious as organic foods.[177] It's not the one-time exposure but the cumulative exposure to chemicals over time that makes one susceptible to lifestyle diseases.

I think that the more the public demands cleaner and healthier methods of cultivating foods, there will be more choices available, everywhere. The food supply will follow the food demand.

CONVENTIONAL PROCESS

Let's look a little more closely at what "conventional food" means. Conventionally grown food begins this way. Manufacturers think, *Let's find a way to produce as much food as possible. It doesn't matter if it's really healthy or not. Let's just feed a lot of people. To keep the nasty bugs away, let's produce truckloads of insecticides and fly planes that drench the food with diabolical chemicals. When people get sick, it's okay; we have a medical system that can treat those problems. Then business will continue to grow and grow.* Look, I'm not saying that there is a conspiracy going on; rather, I am providing an overall picture of our modern food culture and the ramifications of big businesses choosing efficiency and profit over safety and optimum nutrition and health.

Conventional agriculture uses all of the wrong methods and substances. It changes, twists, warps, and modifies the way food should be. It's the synergistic effects that matter, not just one or two bad ingredients over one meal. Conventional food is sponsored by some pretty powerful businesses and it's not going away without a grassroots rally among those of us healthnuts who simply want to live well and be healthy by choice.

HEALTHNUTS...

- Avoid conventionally grown foods that were exposed to any chemicals.
- Purchase local conventional food without chemicals.
- Avoid conventionally grown, GM foods at all costs.

ECONOMICALLY MOTIVATED ADULTERATION

Dead food is just the beginning. Have you heard of EMA? Economically motivated adulteration (EMA) of food is a real problem in our modern society that has negatively influenced nations across the world.[178] Essentially, EMA is a fancy term for food fraud, in which seemingly healthy products like fish, tea, lemon juice, maple syrup, and spices are so recreated via chemical means that they no longer have the health properties of the original product.[179] They are fraudulent because they are fake food—they aren't what they claim to be. Fake food is a disruptor of our normal metabolic state that God created for our bodies. Instead of using fuel for energy, it becomes a leak for toxic gases. Fake food does not fuel healthy bodily function. Fake food fuels toxicity. It is not helpful but actually harmful. If we think about it in these terms, it may help you shift your mind-set for investing in healthier foods that nourish your body. If we love ourselves, we would only want to put goodness into our bodies. Buy the whole, real foods rather than some manufactured artificial version. (More on whole, real foods in Part Four!)

LIVING HEALTHY FOR OTHERS

I often see families at grocery or wholesale clubs buying healthier food items for their kids. They want the best for them. They will go above and beyond to make sure their kids are healthy—but then don't make healthy food choices for themselves! There is often a gap between knowing what is healthy and doing what is healthy. However, it's the doing that produces the health results!

Suppose you were caught on board an airplane with a drastic change in cabin pressure. The pressure drops and there is no oxygen left. Holding your breath you reach for the air mask next to your child. In the process of grabbing the air mask and placing it on your child you lose consciousness and pass out. It's no wonder the airlines say that before you mask someone else, make sure you use your own mask first. So when shopping for food, why would parents provide the best for their children but not take care of themselves?

One of my colleagues wrote a book about his relationship with his father prior to his father's early death from improper nourishment. Heartbroken, my friend went on a mission to not make the same mistake. Even better, he decided to help others not make that same mistake, either. Today, he has a vision to help people with their health by educating doctors to heal their patients with the benefits of a preventive lifestyle.

But you don't have to be a doctor to be a part of this healthnut movement! Choose to eat real food, not just for yourself, but because you want to be around to help others. You are of much value to the world. You have gifts, talents, and insights that will contribute to a better planet. Of course, eating is only one component of health and lifestyle, but it is nonetheless a vital component! Stay away from all forms of toxic foods including GMOs, processed foods, and conventional foods and you are well on your way to overcoming OB and living a long and healthy life.

HEALTHNUTS...

- Avoid fake food to age slowly and for maximum vitality.
- Avoid fake food for optimal metabolism and weight management.
- Avoid fake food for maximum immune system protection and disease risk reduction.

11

HEALTHNUT OVERLOADS

Yum! I love to eat healthy, real food, including snack foods. This may surprise you, but healthnuts enjoy tasteful snacks as much as anyone! My only challenge is that if I like something that is healthy and tastes really good, I may eat too much of it because it feels so healthy!

VALENTINE'S DAY DINNER DELIGHT

For example, during one Valentine's Day, my wife prepared a delicious dinner. We had succulent minted sockeye salmon loaded with omega-3 fatty acids for healthy brain function, lightly steamed spinach with a touch of olive oil for heart support, and freshly pressed vegetable juice for highly absorbable vitamins and minerals. The juice included beets for blood cleansing, kale and spinach for immune support, carrots for additional antioxidants, and fresh lemon for cleaning and increased blood alkalinity. Although dessert was next, I'd already eaten the best part of the meal.

My wife got up from the table and took the freshly baked gluten-free brown rice cherry coconut crumble pie out of the oven. She set the hot pie down on the table and its smell filled the house. She also made a nice coconut honey whip to go on top. My eyes widened, my mouth watered, and my tongue sparked with exuberance. She started by taking a piece for herself, enjoying every bite—and then brought her plate to the kitchen. Unfortunately, I did not follow suit. I gobbled the rest of the entire pie and didn't feel a thing, at first. I remember a little voice that told me to stop indulging on about the third piece. I ignored it. That sound was my wife—she proceeded to tell me about the ten tablespoons of coconut oil she put in the pie!

What? Ten tablespoons?

I know coconut oil is good for you, but not 200+ grams of saturated fat in one sitting! Suddenly, my mind went to work. This was additional fat content on top of the fat I ate during the regular course meal. What was supposed to be a better-for-you pie became a toxic bomb in my stomach. As I sat in a chair feeling achy about fifteen minutes later, blood rushed through my stomach trying to digest the onslaught of food I'd gorged myself on.

I went to bed in pain and eventually fell asleep. Suddenly, I awoke in the middle of the night feeling like I was going to throw up the entire pie. I groaned and moaned, and just could not get comfortable. I threw off the blankets and rushed into the bathroom. My body chilled and coconut-infused sweat seeped out of my pores. Thoughts raced through my mind that the coconut oil was trying to find a way out of my skin. I yelled to my wife to get me a glass of water. Thankfully, she was kind enough to bring me a huge glass along with two digestive enzymes. I gulped down the water along with one of the digestive enzymes. (Yes, in this case I chose to go for extra supplemental support.) I made my way back to the bed and, thankfully, my stomach settled down.

The next morning, everything seemed fully digested. The big lesson I learned is that even if something is good for you, it can become quite disastrous if taken to extremes. Your portion can become a poison. What God made for good can turn bad if we over-indulge.

I wish I could say this experience was a once in a lifetime lesson, but there have unfortunately been many times where I've forgotten my past mistakes and suffered for it. However, I remind myself that it's not about the occasional mistakes: it's about making the right decisions to consistently eat the best foods and stay balanced.

THE CHAMP TOXIN: OVEREATING

Let's explore the champion of toxins. The premier toxin, overeating, is not a direct consumable but applies to any food. To eliminate OB, you have to remove the interference that disallows your body to properly and more effectively eliminate toxins. One of the best ways to do this is to avoid the most toxic foods that contribute to the sludge along with healing the body using the appropriate amount of targeted nutrition. But another way to do this is to simply avoid overeating! Keep in mind that no pill or potion will do the trick. Your "pill" is found on your plate, in your bowl, or in a glass. Although there are many toxins in our world, healthnuts live by the secrets that keep them from overeating on a regular basis. Even if it is a real food, a healthful ingredient can become toxic if overconsumed.

COMMON CAUSES

Overeating the wrong foods is common and is caused by many factors. There are connections between overeating, OB, and addictions to other harmful substances, such as alcohol. It is also hypothesized that chemicals do not cause medical disorders—rather, OB does.[180] However, there are associated links between OB and higher levels of chemical toxins. How can this be? Those who struggle with OB may have a poor function for properly detoxifying toxins such as BPA, which is found in plastics. These toxins, in turn, may disrupt the appropriate hunger-signaling mechanisms that exacerbate the overeating habit, further contributing to OB.

Additionally, medical research reports indicate that hormones such as ghrelin and leptin signal satiety or hunger to the brain.[181] When the body does not respond to these chemical messengers, there is an increase in food consumption, accompanied with weight gain. This is why it's so much easier to maintain a healthy weight once you reach homeostasis, that is, your set range of healthy weight, instead of struggling with the ups and downs of the diet cycle that often prompts us to overeat post-dieting, which numbs our body's natural communication signal that says, "enough!" That normal health communication between the gut and brain is disrupted by toxic foods or by improper digestion.

It's important to focus on the key point that your gut should signal to your brain when you are full. It may take about twenty minutes for this to occur while you eat. That's why you should consider eating slowly and chewing your food. We're all rushed in our modern, fast-paced world, but be mindful of your eating habits. If you've thrown off the proper brain and gut signaling, you're not getting the critical messages that you're really full, which will contribute to the overeating cycle.

HEALTHNUTS...

- Understand eating too much of a good thing may be harmful.
- Drink pure water to reduce some of the toxic effects of overindulgence.
- Reduce health interferences such as toxic food, toxic pills, and toxic emotions.

PREVENTING OVERINDULGENCE

What are conventional methods of stopping the overeating cycle? Health researchers demonstrate self-weighing, food journaling, and other associated forms of dietary monitoring are often employed to combat overeating.[182] These may work to some degree, but you'll have to employ something you can't outsmart too easily.

To avoid overindulgence, one of the best tips is to eat meals at least three hours prior to going to bed. If you eat closer to bedtime, the blood rushes to your gut and causes your heart to race and brain to activate. Some of you may like to have a little snack at night, but if you can avoid it and eat a bigger breakfast in the morning, your metabolism will thank you.

Healthnuts control their eating habits, especially at night. People who go to sleep at the optimal 9–10 p.m. timeframe should stop eating about at 6–7 p.m. I understand that sometimes your work schedule may require a later supper, but if at all possible, it's best to avoid the habit of eating late. Remember that sometimes a "munchy" feeling in the evening might actually be dehydration. Try drinking water, tea, or fresh-juiced vegetables instead of eating a snack.

We live in a culture that prizes overeating. Whether it's football tailgaters or weekend parties, we are mesmerized by the food buffet mentality. Just visit a restaurant. At most modern restaurants, the portions are enough for two people—or a small elephant. What's with Americans that we value quantity over quality?

BRAIN TALK

Clinical trials reveal that eating too much of any variety of food in one meal may contribute to overeating as well.[183] According to Yale endocrinologist

Dr. Robert Sherwin, white processed sugar is linked to shutting off signaling mechanisms in your brain, so you'll keep eating the wrong foods.[184] If you simplify your diet to more real, basic, whole foods you may be tempted to eat less. This is a good temptation! Researchers demonstrate that fewer food choices often leads to lower food consumption.

If you struggle with your weight, it's best to learn what causes the overeating to occur rather than just attempting to overcome your overeating through willpower alone. You may realistically have a health or emotional issue that causes addictive overeating behavior. There are other factors such as dining out, the environment you live or work in, access to physical activity, number of stimulants, and even number of snack food temptations on the go, such as those oh-so-tempting vending machines![185] Yet most, if not all, of these challenges can easily be overcome through proper planning, intention, and action. That's why I believe the Healthnut Life is so critical for people. This lifestyle supports maintaining habits that we choose for ourselves, it is health promoting, it combats addictive food behaviors, and it encourages the right support mechanisms.

OUT OF CONTROL

What if the problem is beyond your control or what if you feel you are too far gone to do anything about it? Oftentimes, overeating can be traced to an imbalance in the digestive and absorption processes of the small intestine. It's important to repair the gut first and then you'll have the proper signals. That is, once you remove foods that may cause you digestive difficulties, you'll once again receive the normal "I'm hungry!" and "no more!" signals. If you continue to eat foods that create low-grade systemic inflammation in your body, however, the overweight condition won't change. You'll just be wasting your money and your efforts.

Healthy habits are easy to make but very difficult to maintain for the long term. That is why most people, according to weight management scholars, are able to take the weight off but unable to keep it off.[186] Therefore, the most critical determinant in the long-term success of a balanced healthy weight is the acquisition of healthy behaviors that lead to a healthy lifestyle. And eating healthily is a behavior that will eventually once again provide your body with the appropriate signaling and nourishment to activate your gut and brain communication. This balanced set point of your ideal "you" is totally possible no matter what challenges you've faced in the past. That's a healthnut promise!

HEALTHNUTS...

- Try to eat no later than three hours prior to sleeping.
- Eat slowly to allow time for hunger signals to slow or stop.
- Chew food thoroughly for maximum digestion.

HEALTHNUT FOREIGN: THREE FOREIGN TOXINS

FOREIGN TOXIN #1: FAKE MEATS

The first foreign toxin is fake meat. Healthnuts won't clog their livers with toxins released from fake or unhealthy processed meats because these meats are virtually indigestible. The main source of fake meats is grain-fed cattle. Interestingly, cows are not even meant to eat grains! It increases their fat content and those grains, which often contain GMOs, are passed along to you. Sometimes clever (but deceptive) marketers will label meats as having been "fed a vegetarian diet." Vegetarian still means corn, soy, or other potential GMO grains. Is this ideal? It's been known for quite some time that not feeding corn to animals makes them lighter, leaner, and overall healthier.[187]

I recently called a farmer to inquire about their raw dairy. Initially he said everything was raw and pasture-raised, but later during the conversation, he mentioned that they feed a mixture of some grains and artificial vitamins to the cattle. The practice of feeding cattle artificial grains and synthetic vitamins is typical. If you do choose to eat meats, eat meat from grass-fed cattle. Unfortunately, grass-fed meat is generally more difficult to find and much more expensive in unconventional grocery stores or local farmers markets.

CLA FAT

Fake meats are nutritionally deprived as well. Fake meats do not have the conjugated linoleic acid (CLA) content that healthy grass fed meats have.[188]

CLA is responsible for helping you to eliminate unhealthy fat in your body. For over thirty years, research supports the benefits of the fatty acid profile of meats from grass-fed animals versus over-consuming meats from grain-fed animals.[189] Researchers contend that eating a larger portion of grain-fed meats may contribute to a similar nutrient profile as a small amount of grass-fed meats. Theoretically, that means we need to eat *more* grain-fed meat to achieve the same nutrient profile. However, wouldn't that defeat the purpose of not overeating?

The CLA content that is gained in consuming smaller portions of grass-fed meats is important for burning fat. That's why weight-loss programs will often recommend foods with high CLA content or will recommend CLA as a dietary supplement. Fake meats, however, don't have the higher levels of CLA and are prone to adding unhealthy saturated fat instead of adding CLA, which is fat burning. This is just one example of the chemical difference in fake meats. There are many other compounds in fake meats that are harmful as well.

HEALTHNUTS...

- Avoid any grain- or soy-fed meats including farm-raised fish, chicken, beef, or turkey.
- Only use grass-fed and grass-finished meats (ask your provider!).
- Avoid drinking milk or other non-organic dairy products from grain-fed cattle.

NITRITES

Healthnuts replace nitrites with real nutritional options. Nitrites are very toxic and have imposed limits of what can be used in the processing of the meat. However, no amount is healthy if you're a healthnut. Any processed lunchmeats or ballpark hot dogs will contain unhealthy nitrites (not to be confused with nitrates) as a meat preservative. Is it a coincidence that researchers are exploring links between processed meats and colorectal cancer and other inflammatory bowel cancers?[190]

Contrast these meats with fresh poultry and meats that are processed naturally and demonstrate some level of protective support against all forms of colorectal cancers through reducing risk of cancer. Once again, the colon is the gateway from mouth and stomach to elimination. Could this toxic sludge putrefy the colon, stopping the effectiveness of the liver and other metabolic functions whose decline contribute to OB?

So, let's explore nitrites in a little more detail to see why they are really harmful. During the cooking process, nitrosamines are formed (a toxic carcinogen) from the nitrites. Nitrites will construct free radicals that lead to oxidation (or rusting) of your cells and body. That's why you may have heard a lot about getting more antioxidants to combat the free radicals in your body. However, no amount of antioxidant consumption will protect you if you regularly ingest an abundance of nitrite chemicals.

Nitrites go beyond digestive and typical OB issues. There is even some preliminary evidence out of China that women who consume nitrites are much more susceptible to thyroid cancer, which may in effect be an underlying contributor to OB.[191] Did you know that thyroid problems are one of the most searched-for medical conditions on the Internet? The demand for thyroid solutions confirms what I've found in consulting clinical practices: a healthy thyroid plays a big role in escaping the clutches of OB for life.[192]

BALLPARK DELIGHTS

How easy is it to avoid nitrites in everyday life? Let me give you an extended example. I used to love to go to the ballpark when I was younger. I looked forward to eating those ballpark dogs. They were juicy and incredible—even if they were five dollars apiece. That investment, however, pays poor dividends. So many of us are duped into believing that just one unhealthy hot dog is okay, just one unhealthy this, one unhealthy that. Healthnuts understand it's not okay. It's always best to find substitutes. There are plenty of safe hot dogs that don't contain all of the chemical toxins. What is the value of your health? Would you pay a dollar more for a healthier hot dog to avoid a $50,000+ surgery? Imagine the savings to healthcare globally by implementing even just *one* of these suggestions.

A number of years ago, I worked with the president of a company who used to say that he had a dangerous colleague whose personality was nice on the outside, but inwardly would "kill you and eat your children." Well, nitrites may look good packaged in that ballpark dog on the outside, but they will kill you and eat your children's insides. In other words, you may want to think twice about that succulent hot dog or those grease-splashed bacon strips on your sandwich. Most importantly, stay away from processed meats and nitrites.

HEALTHNUTS...

- Avoid cured, smoked, or preserved meats.
- Use only hormone- and antibiotic-free fresh or frozen grass-fed meats.
- Avoid ball game hot dogs—bring your own snacks.

FOREIGN TOXIN #2: HYDROGENATED FATS

The second foreign toxin is hydrogenated fat. Healthnuts know hydrogenated fats, including trans fats, are akin to suicide. Hydrogenated or trans fats are hardened and processed. The purpose of these fake fats is to preserve and add firmness to foods such as margarine or vegetable shortening. They will absolutely destroy your arteries because they do not produce free-flowing blood like healthier saturated fats such as coconut oil will do. Although hydrogenated fats are unsaturated, they are not healthy. They will increase the LDL-carrying particle "container" for cholesterol in your body and triglycerides while decreasing good HDL.[193]

This is one of the cases where dietary consumption of an unnatural fat will negatively influence your cholesterol and the lipoprotein transporter particles (LDL, HDL, etc.). To compound the issue, hydrogenated fats are banned in some areas of the country. What's worse, hydrogenated fats are sometimes cloaked with the term *vegetable oil*. Just because it says "vegetable" in the description does not mean it's healthy. It can actually be harmful! Not only are trans fats and partially hydrogenated fats harmful in terms of OB, they will, short of a healing or miracle, distort and ruin your metabolism for life.[194]

In terms of fats and health, triglyceride and HDL measurements are important numbers for you to be concerned about. Triglyceride measurements actually tell you how much fat is in your blood. Why is this important? Well, if your triglyceride levels are high, you have a large amount of fat in your bloodstream. Excess blood fats will clog your arteries and make it more difficult for your heart to work properly.

The other issue with triglycerides is that you may not utilize that fat for energy. Rather, your body is circulating those fats throughout your system. There is a genetic component that affects the configuration of how much fat you will metabolize and store, but most of your storage capacity for triglyceride will coincide with your lifestyle choices. Even the highly respected *Harvard University Public Health Nutrition* confirms that you were not meant to consume trans fats.[195]

HEALTHNUTS...

- Always avoid obvious and hidden hydrogenated fats.
- Only use heart-healthy unrefined fats such as coconut or avocado oil (if necessary).
- Avoid processed pro-inflammatory vegetable oils (soybean, canola, corn, etc.).

MARGARINE

One specific type of hydrogenated fat is margarine. Healthnuts eliminate synthetic margarine from their diets. I remember back in the 1990s, when margarine became popular—it was huge! Everyone was buying it. I Can't Believe It's Not Butter˙ was one memorable brand of margarine. Because margarine didn't have the saturated fats, cholesterol, or any of the other "bad" ingredients like butter, it was somehow better for you. Advertisers promised "healthy" vegetable oils such as polyunsaturated and monounsaturated fats. Great, right?

Wrong.

I was deluded like everyone else. It just seemed natural to slap the fake butter on my toast or bagel in the morning. Immediately, those trans fat tentacles began their toll on my physique. Just a short time after my twenty-first birthday, I awoke from a nap with chest pains. Talk about a rude awakening! This scary experience was one of the warning signals that started me on the path to question my lifestyle behaviors and study the science and art of health, exercise, and nutrition.

Margarine was promoted on the assumption that butter is high in cholesterol and saturated fats, which in turn will increase your bad LDL particles and make you fat. This is erroneous information. Fats do not necessarily make you fat, just like consuming dietary cholesterol does not necessarily increase your blood cholesterol levels.

The real question is not how much butter are you consuming, but what does the lining of your blood vessels actually look like, how many LDL particles do you have, and how many are carrying your cholesterol to the wrong places throughout your body? The takeaway is that the vegetable oils found in margarine and other such products are the most problematic of any oils and increase the risk factors for major cardiovascular diseases.

CHOLESTEROL CHECK

Since it's a matter of such concern to many health-conscious eaters, let's take a look at some cholesterol considerations:

1. Cholesterol is necessary. Cholesterol is used for proper hormone function. Dietary cholesterol is not the same as blood cholesterol. That's been the big problem with all of this talk about cholesterol being bad for you. There is not one study that conclusively proves that high cholesterol leads to a shorter lifespan compared to those who have lower cholesterol. In fact, there is no conclusive proof that having high cholesterol equals more heart attacks and a shorter life span.

This fact is further detailed in Dr. Sinatra and Dr. Bowden's book *The Great Cholesterol Myth*. The book provides a review of why cholesterol is not the enemy, along with several other myths and facts surrounding the benefits of cholesterol.[196] I'm not saying you should have abnormally high rates of cholesterol or not be concerned about your individual lipoprotein particle size levels (LDL, HDL, etc.). What I am saying, however, is to take everything into consideration because the cause may not be what you think!

2. Hydrogenated vegetable oils are not healthy. They are harmful. They increase heart disease risks. You will find these vegetable oils used in many products and restaurants. If you go to a local Indian restaurant, for example, make sure they do not use hydrogenated vegetable oils in their food

preparation. I've experienced this during business trips where I'll fall in love with some foods that contain exceptionally healthy ingredients such as turmeric or other healthy spices, only to find out they use unhealthy vegetable oils!

In one study analyzing trans fats in a high-fat diet, hydrogenated trans fat vegetable oils appear responsible for oxidative stress, insulin resistance, and obesity, along with chronic inflammation.[197] These health risk factors contribute to a toxic liver and ultimately increase risk for cardiovascular disease. No matter how much healthy food you consume, if you eat these toxic hydrogenated foods, you'll overload your system.

3. Margarine is synthetic—a product of changing the chemical structure of the fat to the point that it creates a new fat. You may have heard that plastic bottles contaminate liquids with BPA, which is toxic to your body. In fact, you'll probably see more and more products that claim to be BPA-free because of the movement toward eco-friendly sustainability.

Did you know that BPA is only one toxin and that there are thousands of other toxins that may be connected to your foods as well? Margarine is one such "other toxin" that will increase the risk for cardiovascular disease through inflammation because it's not natural to the body.[198] You better believe it's not butter, or anything real, for that matter.

USE REAL BUTTER

You may or may not like dairy. I am not a big fan of dairy myself as it's never really worked for me, but I know that some people thrive off of real butter. If you need to use butter, use real raw butter that is not homogenized or pasteurized and contains all of the beneficial fat-soluble vitamins, minerals, and enzymes. In this case, it is of course critical that it comes from healthy cows or goats.

According to a report published in the *Journal of Dairy Science*, butter that is produced from cows that graze on pasture contain higher nutritional properties.[199] In effect, the higher concentration of better-for-you dairy properties may reduce risk of forming of fatty plaques in your arteries, as well. This is a somewhat controversial topic; I've heard some experts claim dairy is critical to the diet while others claim that it is harmful. Some studies indicate that butter may be a healthier diet choice, while others demonstrate a higher animal fat diet is a cardiovascular risk factor. Personally, I think it depends on the individual biochemistry, genetics, and epigenetics of the individual.

HEALTHNUTS...

- Avoid margarine or alternative, margarine-like products.
- Use real butter from grass-fed cattle (if required or desired).
- Use ghee as a lower saturated fat alternative to butter (if required or desired).

FOREIGN TOXIN #3: FOOD ADDITIVES

FOOD COLORANTS AND DYES

The third foreign toxin is food additives. Yes, healthnuts die at the hand of their addictions to food dyes. Food dyes have a long and colorful history. Produced from petroleum, they used to be manufactured from coal tar. Now, they're ubiquitous. Turn over your favorite bubble gum and you might find the colors yellow, blue, and red with a number beside them. Or better yet, go to the boxed cereal aisle in the grocery store and you'll see all types of color boxes of cereal. Many of those cereals are not only loaded with sugar, as previously mentioned, but with food colorings and dyes as well. And in numerous studies, these dyes caused adverse health effects. There are other animal studies that show cancer formation from other related toxicity and gene alterations.[200]

It doesn't just stop with food. Colorants are also used in many skin, hair, and nail care products. One chemical common in skin products, titanium dioxide, has been linked to health hazards.[201] These contaminants are absorbed into your skin, just as if you were consuming them. They go right into your bloodstream and manipulate your cells and glands. If it's bad for your stomach, it's equally horrific for your skin. Many of these cancer-causing food colorings are in your most widely used pharmaceutical products as well. Look at the labels. They are full of these inexpensive chemicals. It's just as bad to apply them externally as to ingest them internally.

Even worse, I've seen synthetic colorants in dietary supplements! Recently, I reviewed some literature on an amazing dietary supplement. Though it was very beneficial in preclinical trial research, the supplement had harmful chemicals on the ingredient label. Why would they include them? Because additives are inexpensive and cheap synthetic chemicals or hydrogenated ingredients provide lubrication for the manufacturing of these products. But is it worth reducing some health hazards if it only serves to create other health hazards?

Food companies should target more natural products with truly natural ingredients. Invest resources in the discovery and manufacturing of natural colorants. Natural food colorants, such as anthocyanins found in fruits or vegetables, are a much better option.[202] Hopefully the technology to extract these natural dyes will progress to the point of such ease that it will erase the use of synthetic materials.

HEALTHNUTS...

- Avoid personal or food products containing food dyes and colorants.
- Substitute natural non-toxic ingredients and products.
- Avoid other products with food additives, such as dietary supplements.

MONOSODIUM GLUTAMATE (MSG)

Another major additive is MSG. MSG is basically a concentrated form of salt that directly contributes to OB. Healthnuts resist MSG (whether called MSG or any of its alternative names). MSG is a salt of glutamic acid, a non-essential amino acid. It is used as a flavoring additive and combined with many types of foods. However, some studies correlate MSG to allergic reactions and possible neurotransmitter dysfunction, since glutamates play a role in brain function. MSG is notorious for being added to dishes at oriental restaurants. However, MSG can be found in almost any restaurant, combined with hydrolyzed protein, yeast extracts, and other forms of protein. These proteins are indigestible or non-absorbable by the body and cause low-grade inflammation leading to autoimmune dysfunction in your body. MSG is hidden in sauces and is mixed with other grocery store stock items. Some of the products are soups—that are often claiming to be natural or healthy! There are lists of ingredients that replace the term "MSG" with something else or are combined with other ingredients and seasonings.[203]

Did you also know that MSG is used in labs to induce obesity in rats?[204] Surely that indicates its dangerous link to weight gain! Another study, reported in *Physiology & Behavior*, found that rats consuming MSG-added trans fats, which are the worst kinds to mix, experienced abnormally high levels of cholesterol and their short-term memory was impaired.[205] Now, do you want any MSG or trans fats? I don't think so—and I'm sure you'd like to also keep your memory and cholesterol levels normal.

That's one of the reasons you have to be extra cautious when you see words like "natural flavors" on the back of your food product's label. There may be nothing natural about the flavorings. The marketing term may be a disguise for MSG, instead of truly natural flavors like those manufactured from oranges or pineapples. In these cases, MSG may not be directly listed on the label because it is not directly added. However, it is mixed with other ingredients. You have to be aware when you see a product advertised as having no added MSG—because the MSG may be mixed in with the other ingredients![206]

HEALTHNUTS...

- Request no sauce and no MSG at restaurants.
- Use natural seasoning or real pink rock salt instead (without overdoing the salt).
- Avoid store products with MSG or MSG derivatives labeled.

HEALTHNUT UNREAL: THREE UNREAL TOXINS

UNREAL TOXIN #1: TOXIC SUGAR

ADULTEROUS FRUCTOSE

The first unreal toxin is toxic sugar. Healthnuts only consume natural forms of sugar. Natural sugar's unnatural, broken-down form, fructose, is very harmful. Fructose is a common sugar found in fruits, which is sweeter than glucose (another form of sugar), but which is toxic when not surrounded by fiber, as it is in fruit. University of Oxford researchers studied corrupted forms of fructose and their contribution to OB.[207] After the study was published, one of the co-authors of the study clarified in an interview that fruit fructose is "fine."[208] But fructose consumed on its own, not with fruit, is not fine! Fructose is found to increase insulin resistance, metabolic disruption, and altogether increases aging. It also has an addictive effect according to fructose researcher Dr. Robert Lustig.[209] Even worse, fructose is implicated in obesity and fatty liver disease.[210]

If you are struggling with your weight or body fat, fat is not your enemy. Sure, unhealthy fats like certain types of saturated and polyunsaturated fats that I've discussed are best avoided. However, healthy fats are beneficial. The real problem is fructose. Fructose is not friendly for your metabolism. Fructose raises your blood sugar and blood pressure. Fructose depletes your metabolism by making it more difficult for you to burn fat. You actually burn carbs and the fat stays. Worse, the fructose is converted and stored as fat.[211]

A MINDFUL EFFECT

The other problem is that fructose plays tricks with your brain. A recent study in *JAMA* found that fructose does not block the reward and appetite areas in the brain. Compare this with glucose sweeteners that will shut off the reward and appetite region as a natural hunger control mechanism.[212] In other words, a glucose sweetener will signal to your body when enough is enough. A fructose sweetener, however, will always demand more, and more, and more!

Although fructose is found in natural fruits, there it is coupled with fiber. If you strip the fiber from the fruits, it becomes merely a sugar rush. There are some healthy foods that contain natural fructose, like raw honey. The difference is that when you consume raw honey, you only take a small amount at a time. The purpose of this dose of honey is to sweeten a bit of food and increase B vitamins and propolis, which supplies excellent energy and is a great immune booster. Other than that, there is no reason to consume large amounts of honey. If heated, the fructose in the honey will also have negative effects on the body. So as you've already learned, just because something is good for you, doesn't mean you should eat a lot of it.

HEALTHNUTS...

- Understand the difference between real and unreal fructose.
- Eliminate the toxic forms of fructose without the fiber.
- Use special nutrients in very small amounts (raw honey for vitamins or energy).

HIGH FRUCTOSE CORN SYRUP

If you thought your only problem was fructose, think again. Fructose's evil twin is high fructose corn syrup (HFCS). HFCS was invented in the 1960s and introduced to the US diet in 1975. This is about the time these artificial sweeteners were really ramped up on the market. The purpose was to make food really, really cheap. HFCS is so inexpensive to produce that it is now in nearly every food that allows it. Whether it's HFCS or fructose, it has the potential to, over time, alter your gut bacteria. If your gut bacterium is negatively unbalanced, you are less likely to have a healthy metabolism because you are not properly assimilating your foods.[213]

High fructose corn syrup is implicated in many weight problems. Much of this begins with the toxic accumulation in the liver leading to fatty liver disease.[214] Your liver will make sure HFCS is stored as fat versus used for energy. The liver is also responsible for healthy hormone balance and detoxifying excess estrogen that leads to belly fat. An unhealthy liver impedes your ability to achieve your ideal weight. Worse, HFCS also triggers to your brain to eat more HFCS so that you can't escape the OB cycle!

In a review of numerous studies, HFCS was found to increase the risk of obesity in children.[215] It is very hard on insulin levels in the body. The production process for this synthetic sweetener requires the toxic element mercury as well. HFCS is unnatural and produces unnatural results. It's also involved in many supplement products including protein powders and meal bars.

I am always surprised when I meet with a few health professionals that still recommend weight-loss and detoxification products that are composed of high fructose corn syrup. HFCS is also hidden in many products—undisclosed—so it's sometimes difficult to tell if it's included. Supposedly healthy foods (such as salad dressings) are some of the worst offenders. You think you are making a healthier choice, but it's not the fat in the dressing—it's the sugar. You'll see gimmick marketing hype "low fat" or "no fat." Yeah, but it is high sugar! That sugar leads to more fat in your body and organs.

HEALTHNUTS...

- Avoid high fructose corn syrup (HFCS) products.
- Use only natural sweeteners in small amounts.
- Always consume some fiber with sweetened foods.

UNREAL TOXIN #2: TOXIC SWEETENERS

If sugar is really so harmful, it's hard to imagine that artificial sweeteners would be even worse—but they are! Healthnuts always pass on those little pink and blue packets. I recently went out with a friend who was concerned about her health—and was surprised when she reached for the little pink packet. That is really a micro-death packet. That pink wrapper looks really innocent, but inside is slow, chemical poison. It's funny that people who promote a healthy lifestyle will still use the little blue and pink packets as if their immune systems will fight off any negative effects. They don't realize that, inevitably, the toxicity will show up somewhere in their bodies.

In existence since the late nineteenth century, artificial sweeteners such as saccharin have gone through a series of labeling challenges. What you have to remember is that anything artificial already violates the principle eating only real and natural food. If it is chemically altered, there are going to be deleterious effects, whether or not they have yet been discovered.

ARTIFICIAL ASPARTAME

Although there are many artificial sweeteners, let's look at a specific artificial flavoring called aspartame. Aspartame is much sweeter than raw sugar. Although it is listed as "safe" in almost one hundred countries, it is not safe! It is very toxic and harmful. What's confusing for consumers is there were some previous studies that suggested the benefits of aspartame for maintaining a healthy body weight.[216] Companies likely used this information to explain why they should include aspartame in their products.

When it comes to something artificial, research can change its opinion over time. The problem with these studies is they only take into account reduced appetite, not the side effects of consuming aspartame over the long term. Aspartame can be stored and used in the body and is not excreted like other sweeteners. It is linked to increasing risks for cancers, weight gain, diabetes, and neurological damage to the brain.[217] Aspartame actually creates more of a dependence on sugar and non-artificial sweeteners.[218]

When I was bodybuilding, I used to drink this protein shake that contained aspartame. I was trying to gain as much mass as possible and had at least three shakes per day. That pink flavor that I loved was the cloak for the aspartame hidden inside. I gulped thousands of these shakes in my late teens and early twenties. No wonder I had gastrointestinal issues for so many years. I was deceived into thinking that my external appearance was the determination of how healthy I was. What a lie.

Just because you look good on the outside doesn't mean you're healthy. That's why some models look incredibly thin, but if you were to take their body fat percentage, you would find they are 50% fat! See, when we're young in our teens and twenties, we think thirties or forties are a long way off. Suddenly we find ourselves in the throes of aging as our thirties creep into our forties. Then we are in the fifties going to sixties, and we wish we had begun sooner. By the time we are in our seventies and eighties, it's often way too late: the damage is done. Instead of living with vitality in our latter years, we are diseased, debilitated, and depressed.

That's why, starting now, we all need to be really inquiring about what's in our food today. The reality is that the very item you believe is healthy may contain aspartame or a similar ingredient that will cause characteristic cell death.

HEALTHNUTS...

- Avoid all foods with aspartame and hidden sources of aspartame.
- Avoid diet foods that claim to be healthy but have toxic ingredients like aspartame.
- Use natural sweeteners instead such as real fruits (with the fiber).

SUCRALOSE

I would be remiss if I didn't mention the popular sweetener Sucralose. Healthnuts aren't fooled by large company endorsements for synthetic sugar substitutes. In the US there are seven sweeteners that are approved by the government. They include Acesulfame K, Aspartame, Luo Han Duo Fruit Extract, Neotame, Saccharin, Stevia, and Sucralose.[219]

Unfortunately, government approval does not guarantee safety or health, and both sucralose and aspartame in particular may cause problems for you. Sucralose, whose brand name is Splenda, is a sugar replacement. It has zero calories and no effects on blood sugar. It is artificial, manufactured in a lab. The diet industry is notorious for promoting Sucralose. I've seen it on TV commercials. However, contrary to some media opinion, Sucralose is shown to not reduce appetite.[220] Sucralose also alters gut microflora, further increasing the propensity for intestinal permeability or "leaky gut," the condition mentioned in chapter 9.[221] This effect contributes to a wide range of food intolerance susceptibility and potentially autoimmune reactivity in your body.

In other words, that short-term weight loss you'll experience by using these artificial sweeteners is exchanged for long-term intestinal destruction. If you can't properly assimilate your food, where do you think the food goes? Into your bloodstream, producing more toxins in your body, stressing your liver, and thus repeating the weight gain, or body fat storage, process. It's much easier to avoid this cycle by removing artificial sweeteners from your diet.

HEALTHNUTS...

- Avoid Sucralose as an added sweetener.
- Are not duped by Sucralose "diet foods" claiming weight loss benefits.
- Avoid Sucralose to maintain a healthy gut bacterial balance.

SUGAR ALCOHOLS

Sugar alcohols are a special carbohydrate known as a polyol. Chemically, it looks like a cross between sugar and alcohol, from which it derives its name, "sugar alcohol." Sugar alcohols have been used in various products, especially in those that promote weight loss.

A report on artificial sweeteners from Mayo Clinic indicates that sugar alcohols are beneficial in terms of weight loss and diabetes.[222] However, they are very hard on the gut, and if consumed in excess, will influence blood sugar negatively. The benefits derived from the sugar alcohol, which does not influence blood sugar as rapidly as normal sugar, will unfortunately disrupt your ability to assimilate nutrients.

Unfortunately, the real, healthy sugars are not promoted like manufactured sugars. Sugar alcohols are very popular in food bars, for example. Companies will show that their products are low in sugar. That looks great, until you see they are loaded with sorbitol, maltitol, and other -tols that take a toll on your health.

It's true that sugar alcohols normally do not impact blood sugar levels, but they will irritate your digestive system. If you consume them, you may not have high blood sugar increases, but you will have disturbed digestion. That disruption will lead to other problems with nutrient absorption and potential toxicity in the form of a defective immune system. Immune dysfunction is a catalyst for hormone and gland dysfunction. It's a cycle that begins and ends with something unnatural and unreal.

Sugar alcohols are marketed as no-calorie sweeteners. Health diet companies and even high quality health professional formulas may contain these in their products. Quite often, weight-loss products or beverages will use these sugar alcohols as well. You'll reduce your caloric intake, but you'll make it more difficult to keep the weight off in the future. If your gut isn't functioning properly, you'll cause other imbalances—including a weight imbalance! That's why everything begins and ends with your gut and what you put in your mouth. Your long-term health starts with consuming the right foods—and your body will provide you with future benefits.

HEALTHNUTS...

- Avoid sugar alcohols in order to reduce or eliminate digestive difficulties.
- Substitute with natural sweeteners, such as dates.
- Avoid weight-loss products with sugar alcohols (an additive).

UNREAL TOXIN #3: TOXIC BEVERAGES

SODA

Toxic sugar and toxic sweeteners make America's most popular beverage a toxic drink! Regular soda is toxic because of its absurdly high levels of sugar. Healthnuts expunge soda from their diet for maximum weight management. There is a war between soft drink manufacturers and the public interest with the fight against OB, which has become so intense that the manufacturers denounce statements by interest groups, and the interest groups denounce statements by the manufacturers. For example, the Executive Director at the Center for Science in the Public Interest (CSPI) went so far as to claim that the scientific community has finally agreed that "soft drinks are the one food or beverage that's been demonstrated to cause weight gain and obesity."[223]

Even worse, children seem to be the most vulnerable by the onslaught of toxic beverage consumption. A recent study of 319 Mexican-American children in the *Public Health Nutrition Journal* concluded that children who consumed soft drinks had higher rates of obesity versus kids who avoided soft drinks.[224] Of course, it's not just kids who struggle with these sugar-sweetened concoctions. Adults lose out as well. The *American Journal of Clinical Nutrition* published a report from a meta-analysis review of thousands of children and adults, which concluded that sugary drink consumption is directly linked to increases in body mass index and weight gain. The authors point out that there are other dietary and lifestyle factors at play, but the associations with OB are indisputable.[225]

An end-year study in the *Nutrition Journal* of 3,583 children on sugar-sweetened beverage patterns found higher correlations of OB with those who consumed these sugar-sweetened beverages.[226] A smaller scale, six-month randomized study demonstrated increases in all forms of fat and risks for cardiovascular disease and metabolic diseases with the consumption sugar-sweetened beverages.[227]

Advertising contributes to the vast popularity of these toxic beverages. It's well-known that multimedia and even outdoor advertising is connected to buyers' overconsumption, which is linked to OB.[228]

No matter what kind of soda you're drinking; the sugar is enough to kill! There are multiple teaspoons of sugar in each can of soda. Average this out over a year, and soda-drinkers are consuming several boxes of straight sugar. Unfortunately, states have voted down extreme measures of banning or taxing soda.[229] With mounting evidence of its danger, however, that may change in the near future—especially if the public demands it!

DIET SODA

Can you imagine anything worse than soda? Well, there is something: *diet* soda. It goes against conventional marketing wisdom: companies tout diet drinks as a healthier alternative to the traditional, sugar-filled beverages. But these drinks are even more destructive! In a large analysis of over 60,000 women from 1993, researchers reported in the *American Journal of Clinical Nutrition* that diet soda and artificially sweetened beverages increased diabetes risk just as much, if not more, than their sugar-sweetened counterpart.[230]

Essentially, this study proposes that type 2 diabetes risk is directly correlated to OB in the consumption of artificially sweetened beverages.

Diet soda will kill, not from the sugar, but from the sugar substitutes that are actually cell-altering chemicals. Marketers keenly understand the consumer shift from soda to diet soda, and they exploit it. Healthnuts don't drink any diet sodas because they know that it contains toxic, anti-nutrient ingredients that are harmful to their digestive systems. You can't take shortcuts for your health and expect great returns! The dangers of soda and diet soda are not just physical; some new research links soda with depressive and addictive behaviors.[231] It's like caffeine—once you start, it's difficult to stop.

Even sports beverages may contain the unnatural flavorings or sweeteners that will contribute to OB by acting as an anti-nutrients. Often, these sports beverages have just as much sugar as soda. I used to drink these fiber-lacking juices when I was kid. I didn't know any better and, like me, many kids and adults today drink these fake juices without thinking. Even if the labels claim 100% juice, it's not enough! Make sure that the juices you drink contain the insulin-friendly fiber.

HEALTHNUTS...

- Use fresh, cold-pressed or flash pasteurized fruit beverages.
- Use flavored waters (preferably herbal flavored waters).
- Always avoid both regular and diet soda.

CAFFEINE

Healthnuts reduce or eliminate excess caffeine—and yes, that includes coffee! Now, since there's a good chance you're in the half of the world's population who drink a few cups of coffee a day, I ask you at least hear me out. Yes, it's true that coffee and tea are associated with lower risk of type 2 diabetes.[232] And caffeine in its natural form is found in plants, nuts, cherries, and the cocoa bean.[233] But although that may sound great—if it grows on a plant, it's healthy, right?—the way it is processed in the body can be not so great. You see, the caffeine in coffee is processed at a high temperature which strips it of its nutrients, and, like in carbonated soft drinks, dietary supplements, and energy drink products, the amount of caffeine in coffee is unnaturally high, which changes its metabolic and physiological effect. Although some studies point to some beneficial effects, in contrast, larger doses of caffeine are also associated with liver, cardiovascular, and nervous system issues, along with the accompanying anxiety.[234]

Please understand that all raw cacao or cocoa contains at least a small amount of caffeine. Raw products vary, and it is up for debate how much actual caffeine is in each product. You have to check if the caffeine information on the cacao or cocoa product is readily discernable. Others believe the levels of caffeine in raw cacao or cocoa are such a tiny fraction of what you find in coffee or even tea, they have a minimal effect on blood sugar. Furthermore, dietary, unsweetened cacao fed to mice has been shown to have a positive effect on obesity by decreasing the associated inflammation, increasing beneficial gut microbes (although more clinical trials are needed).[235]

So, for example, genuine cacao or cocoa may be fine if consumed in reasonable amounts—good news for those of you who love the chocolate flavor! There are also beneficial polyphenolic flavonols in cacao as well. Watch out, however, because cacao may be mixed with soy, sugar or other unnatural ingredients to make it more palatable. Cocoa also contains numerous phytochemical benefits, such as reducing the risk of cardiovascular disease and hypertension while having a positive effect on OB.[236] However, cocoa may be processed with higher temperatures and solvents which decrease some of the nutritional quality.

I want to emphasize that we are talking about unhealthy amounts of caffeine found in products. Is it any coincidence that a meta-analysis review of numerous studies over a thirty-year period found a positive link between coffee consumption and bladder cancer?[237] It's likely that the amount and form of caffeine is the real problem.

Caffeine acts like a stimulant drug and as a psychoactive chemical, that, when mixed with other substances, creates dependent devotion, much like alcohol.[238] You'll notice that I'm assuming you realized the dangers attached to alcohol consumption. If you're drinking alcohol, you probably know exactly what you're doing to your body. But coffee is a bit more sneaky. Is it healthy or not? I say not.

Caffeine, it has been shown, creates a cocaine-like addiction, further complicating its effect on humans. Although some tout the benefits of preventive antioxidant effectiveness against cancer, caffeine is prone to increase anxiety and sleep disorders.[239] Sleep disorders are also correlated to OB, just as much as alcohol or constant TV watching.[240] So, in effect, although caffeine is not the direct cause of OB, through its tendency to cause sleep disorders, it may also contribute to OB. Caffeine is also a diuretic and increases the risk of dehydration.[241]

Some claim that caffeine may have weight reduction benefits. Other reports, however, show that caffeine has no effect on actual body weight reduction.[242] It stimulates the nervous system and that's why it is considered toxic at high doses. It also creates dependence and potentially adverse side effects.[243] So what happens when you can't consume caffeine or try to go off of it? You have the withdrawal symptoms and may go back to the lifestyle practices that caused weight gain and increased body fat in the first place. Caffeine creates dependence and that is never helpful when trying to create sustainable lifestyle healthy eating practices. Unfortunately, although caffeine does give you a great energy boost, for the above reasons it simply can't be described as entirely healthful.

Companies are also mixing caffeinated coffee with other beverages. The FDA announced in recent years that combining caffeine with other substances, such as alcohol, is unsafe.[244] This should raise the question, what else is unsafe when combined with caffeine? Marketers have also tried to promote "healthier" coffee and teas with little or no caffeine as well. These are better substitutes for any drinks with higher amounts of caffeine. Ideally, though, your drinks should contain no caffeine. A reasonable amount of cacao nibs is not the issue (if you've never eaten a cacao nib, look it up!). The unhealthy, processed mixed drinks and dietary supplements, however, are a huge problem. Natural vitamins, minerals, amino acids, and other nutrients should provide the boost energy you require every day for normal function, not caffeine.

HEALTHNUTS...

- Avoid unhealthy, processed caffeinated beverages.
- Avoid coffees (and only drink low or no caffeine versions if absolutely necessary).
- Drink plenty of fresh water if consuming caffeine.

CONCERNED ABOUT DANGEROUS FOOD YOU MAY BE EATING?
JOIN THE HEALTHNUT COMMUNITY BY VISITING **DRHEALTHNUT.COM**
FOR BONUS TIPS ON HOW TO INCREASE CRAVINGS FOR HEALTHY FOODS.

SCAN TO VISIT DRHEALTHNUT.COM

PART FOUR:

DR. HEALTHNUT REAL

14

HEALTHNUT FOODS

REAL FOODS

When I was younger, I didn't think too much about nutrition. I was always of the mind-set that it was a good thing to get more food for less. At least, that's the message that the media continually pumped to my generation. It was about tasty food for short-term enjoyment rather than quality food for long-term health. I was a sucker (like everyone else following the herd). Then one day I awoke with pain in my chest and realized that the electric surge I experienced should not be happening at twenty-one years of age! How could this be? I lay in my bed and heard a voice that told me to start changing my lifestyle. I believe God was graciously warning me that if I were to continue going down the same familiar path, my life would end a lot sooner than necessary.

Although I didn't make changes overnight, I slowly began taking steps toward more healthful nutrition. I am certainly a far cry from where I need to be today, but I have made some great progress over the years. I believe that you can make improvements, too. You can take the necessary steps for a more healthful life. If you are younger, you can start today and save yourself a lifetime of preventable health struggles. If you are older, don't worry. It's never too late. Consider this: if fruit flies that eat quality nutrition and real food live healthier and longer than the flies that eat toxic food, you, a human, are in much better position than a fruit fly to live with vitality.[245]

155

Healthnuts eat real food. Real food is exactly opposed to its nemesis, its arch-enemy: toxic food. Toxic food is devoid of nutrients and has been altered in some fashion. Real food is something that God has either created or blessed. That doesn't mean it is always a living food. I love living foods. They are probably the largest part of my diet. But real food also consists of healthy meats. Some of you may be vegetarian or vegan and that's great too. It's whatever works with your body—as long as it is real instead of anything artificial.

Real food contains a wide spectrum of vitamins, minerals, antioxidants, phytochemicals, proteins, fats, and complex carbohydrates. I'm talking now about balanced nutrition. This real food principle is contrary to diets that depend on a handful of nutrients or an excess of one specific nutrient. The most effective method of using real foods is to consume the rainbow of fruits and vegetables for added micronutrient prevention and macronutrient fats, proteins, and carbohydrates for bodily fuel and function.

HEALTHNUTS...

- Eat real food for optimal nutritional value and nutrient density.
- Eat real food for cellular health and anti-aging benefits.
- Eat real food for pH balance to reduce the risk of preventable lifestyle diseases.

3 HEALTHY FOOD PRINCIPLES

Healthnuts abide by 3 key food principles for maximum health. To really understand what a healthnut thinks, you need to see how they view real food. These principles apply to any diet types.

HEALTHNUTS...

1. Eat real foods.
2. Eliminate all toxic foods.
3. Eat this way for life.

Now of course, these mean different things to different people, but essentially they are your lifelong guides for lifestyle living. Essentially, healthnuts are less focused on what they *can't* eat than on what they *can* eat! Within these guides, you have to find what works best for you. What is amusing is that there are diets and formulas that emphasize and compare one diet over another. The reality is, everyone is different, so, logically, there cannot be one diet that works best for everybody.

There are vegetarians who strongly believe that what they do is right for them. I myself like to consume small portions of meat, because I believe that's best for my body. Does that mean I should persuade them to eat my way? Absolutely not—they should do what they believe is best for their body! This is the art of health, and I love it for its never-ending, individual-based challenge.

SEASONS OF LIFE

It's ok to eat differently in different seasons of life. To illustrate, I once tried a stint on a vegan diet. I couldn't do it long-term. Other times I consumed a heavy meat diet. That didn't work either. I ended up coming back to a balanced view for my health. Personally, I believe that about 75–85% of our food intake should come from whole foods that are living and 15–25% from real foods such as meats. This is my personal philosophy at this time. That doesn't mean my philosophy will never change. There are different seasons in life. I will adjust my eating plan to fit the changing seasons, just as you will. The main point is that whatever season we are in, we should always consume real foods!

What about athletes? They have different demands for proteins, fats, and carbohydrates—as we've discussed. Should an Olympic swimmer eat a low calorie vegetarian diet? I'm sure it could be done, but it probably wouldn't be to their advantage! Surely they would not long be a champion in their chosen discipline. Some of the diets of Olympians are upwards of 10,000 calories a day!

The number of calories is not what determines "healthy" or "unhealthy." Rather, it's the holistic view that encompasses your whole body and mind that can determine whether you're "healthy" or "unhealthy." Never let a website or fad diet book convince you that you're eating unhealthily. Instead, remember that you're an individual with a unique set of strengths and weaknesses. Consult a holistic health examiner, and make life choices based on where you've been, where you are, and where you'd like to be.

But how do these principles translate into what you're actually going to eat for breakfast, lunch, or dinner this week? Well, let's review the previously mentioned three main categories of real foods, based on these principles.

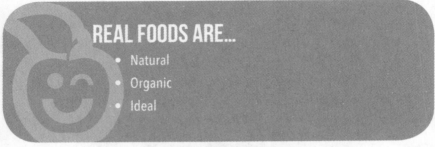

REAL FOODS ARE...
- Natural
- Organic
- Ideal

REAL FOOD #1: NATURAL

NATURAL CONFUSION

Healthnuts choose the right natural foods and avoid the wrong natural foods. Natural is such a widespread term used for so many different parts in the food and nutrition industry. You read, "This chicken is natural and hormone-free" at the local restaurant and wonder, *What does that actually mean?* The FDA states that it is difficult to define a food as "natural" because every food has at least been minimally processed, unless you're the blessed gardener who just eats tomatoes right off the vine.[246]

So, natural may mean without antibiotics or added colors, artificial flavors, or other synthetic substances, or it may not. Chickens can be natural, but only if everything they grazed on was natural. Fruits can be natural but does that mean they were grown in healthy soil? Was the soil sprayed with pesticides, herbicides, or fungicides? Natural food is much better than conventional food, but it is undeniable that the food industry uses the term "natural" in order to sell more products. Advertising veils the real distinction of what's natural, and what's not.

MARKETING NATURAL

Pick a packaged natural product off the shelf and it might contain abnormally high levels of sugar, gluten, and other forms of toxic anti-nutrients or even fake foods! How can this be? One word: marketing.

Many of our communities thrive off of colorful boxes of fake oats with artificial colorings or flavor-enhanced ice promoted by ice cream trucks. That famous ding-dong bell rings in my ears to this day. As a kid, that was the call for a sugar-drenched sweet. I would hear the sounds and my eyes would tear, my chest would pump, and my mouth would water. I would run to my mom and ask for some change or scour the house to find a jar of pennies and count every last one. I would dash outside and line up for my ice cream sandwich. But why did I respond that way? Why did I not understand that this was fake food and was harming my precious internal possessions? One word: marketing. I was programmed just like many other children in the 1980s, with the latest and greatest commercials sandwiched between my favorite cartoons. Fake food brainwashing! Oh, those were the days.

Now, it's a different story. I'm obviously not a kid anymore (at least in my mind), and I've been exposed to the genius behind the low-cost, high-profit, fake food production cycles. Do you really know how much that frosted cream-filled chocolate cake cost to source, manufacturer, and produce compared to what they sell it for? I didn't think that way either when I rode my bike to the convenience store for another round of Ho Hos. I wasn't raised in a family that had the background in nutrition or understanding of health, like some of my colleagues. My parents did the best they could with the knowledge they had available. And I made poor choices of my own volition.

But let's return to one important word. *Marketing*. Like me, have you fallen for the same deception? Just because the package says "natural" does not mean it's healthy for you (or even real, for that matter). At one point, the FDA made a determination that it considered high fructose corn syrup—and we've already covered its dangers!—as natural.[247] "Natural" also allows for toxic pesticides, GMOs, antibiotics, growth hormones, and irradiation as well in some instances. (Doesn't sound very natural, does it?) Each product individually must have its own analysis to determine if it is really healthy for you or not. On top of that, ask yourself whether it is a product that you need at that moment, whether you can wait for it, or—even better—substitute something else in its place!

AUTHENTIC NATURAL

See, natural can be anything we want it to be. Just like beauty, "natural" is only defined by the beholder—or consumer. Sadly, the definition has lost its character, meaning, and austere luster. But we can change that. We can get back to the way it should be. Natural should be just that, "natural," without anything artificially synthetic added and without being processed in any way that detracts from the definition of truly natural.

Let me give you an example that cuts through the confusion and demonstrates what natural food is. A local farmer close to where I live doesn't have a certified organic farm, but has still made the commitment not to use any pesticides, herbicides, fungicides, or any other chemicals on the foods they grow. They use healthy non-GMO seeds during the growing process, as well. They don't skimp on providing the healthiest soil possible for farming their products. The process they use is similar to what is used in Amish country, where farmers use real manure as fertilizer. You know, the stuff that stinks! It's really amazing how something that smells so nasty can transform into a food so healthy. Although not all farmers are like this in Amish country, many abide by the real food growing principles.

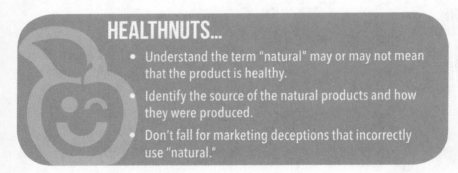

HEALTHNUTS...

- Understand the term "natural" may or may not mean that the product is healthy.
- Identify the source of the natural products and how they were produced.
- Don't fall for marketing deceptions that incorrectly use "natural."

REAL FOOD #2: ORGANIC

Organic is better than natural food because thanks to recent laws, its authenticity is in some way measurable and verifiable, unlike the "natural" label, which can be slapped on just about anything. Organic, in the truest sense, means that the food is grown from healthy seeds, in healthy soil, without the influence of any chemicals or anything artificial. Note that there are different levels of organic: there is 50% organic, 80% organic, and 100% organic. There is even "certified organic," which essentially means that the USDA has vouched for the product. The USDA's certification process is lengthy and quite an investment. The inspectors periodically review and audit select organizations to make sure their organic standards of food growing is up to par.

CHEMICAL ECONOMICS

Our industries glorify pesticides, herbicides, fungicides, and insecticides to our farmers and growers, who end up regularly using damaging chemicals. Why do most of the farmers use chemicals versus growing organically? Many point out that the decision farmers must make whether or not to grow real food simply comes down to an economic consideration: it's more expensive to grow organic food. While this may be true, it is the healthnut's dream that a booming market for organic products will soon lead more and more farmers and growers to decide to grow organic products. As more research comes out, organic food is vindicated again and again. One of the most impacting studies found that although there may not be a significant difference in quality of food, organic foods might reduce exposure to pesticides and antibiotic resistant bacteria.[248]

Healthnuts ought to be cautious, however, of waiting for a pile of studies to agree on what is or is not healthy! What if you eat a specific type of non-organic food and twenty years from now you find it causes cancer? Is it worth it? Go with what makes sense and support how your body was designed to function. Certified organic will always be non-GMO. Also, organic produce at your grocer will begin with the number nine on the label sticker.

HEALTHNUTS...
- Invest in real quality soil versus synthetic soil counterfeits.
- Support farmers and growers who use sustainable farming practices.
- Limit consumption of foods and products with environmental chemicals.

ORGANIC STANDARDS

Frankly, the organic standard has been subjected to marketing abuses. Similar to "natural," the term is now diluted. Certified organic producers are allowed to use low-level grades of organic pesticides. This is confirmed through the National Organic Standards Board that determines which "minimal" pesticides are allowed in production. The problem is, anti-nutrients are introduced and even lead to what is termed by The Cornucopia Institute as "Organic Watergate."[249]

So buyers must beware: just because a food is organic does not necessarily mean it is pesticide-free. A recent analysis by the Canadian Food Inspection Agency found that almost 50% of tested samples of organic fruits and vegetables contained pesticide residues.[250]

Whether or not you agree with accusatory scandals, and although the amounts of what is included in organic products are probably minor compared to conventionally grown food, even trace amounts are enough to warrant the question—why gamble with our lives? What is truly organic? Organic should mean "products that are grown without any harmful anything at any time in any soil." The reality, however, is that stringent definitions are very difficult both to instigate and to implement.

MARKETING ORGANIC

There are some organic and even certified organic products that are not as healthy as some natural products, and vice versa. I may stretch it a bit with this statement, but even certain types of conventionally grown food may be healthier than some certified organic treats. Before you stone me, please allow me to explain in detail. I walked into a regular grocery store recently. I decided to take a stroll down the dreaded middle aisles. (I should add that if you shop at a grocery store you should keep to the outside aisles. That is where the fresh foods and healthy meats are located.)

As I perused the aisles, I came across the natural and organic section. I looked at some of the labels and was horrified. Certified organic cane juice. What is that? Just because it's certified organic it makes it better than regular sugar? Sugar is sugar. Period. This was listed as the top ingredient in the so-called certified organic product. How many people were duped into believing this was good for them because they didn't take the time to check out the product in more detail?

And so, there in the grocery store, I arrived again at the famous nine-letter word. Yes, you guessed it: Marketing. Times have changed, and there is a movement toward healthier food choices, but marketing has not changed. The marketers have just adapted their techniques to include savvy trend analysis coupled with juicy advertising messages that bypass the health of the busy consumer.

REAL ORGANIC

I've seen organic cookies on the shelf as well. My wife is the only one who can make real organic cookies. (OK, you caught me—I do love her cookies.) She uses the healthiest ingredients to make them. I hope you realize it's not about rules and regulations. It's about principle in terms of what you eat. It's best to prepare the food yourself, knowing that the ingredients are real, and not refined, than to guess what's inside someone else's fake concoction.

There are other aspects to organic that are important, including the cultivation practices in organic farming. Organic farming to some degree demonstrates protection of agriculture and biodiversity and even pest control as compared to conventional food growing practices.[251] Organic is about getting back to the farm or local store as much as possible. Sure, big chains can emulate this well. They may partner with farmers and other specialty product manufacturers. We need to question everything and rethink our definitions of what is healthy, what is better for you, and what is not healthy.

I'm changing my definition of the highest level of real food from organic to ideal…as you'll see in the next section.

HEALTHNUTS...

- Understand the differences between certified organic and organic foods.
- Support and use real organic food when possible (not perfect but better).
- Avoid the marketing gimmicks of organic foods that are not healthy.

REAL FOOD #3: IDEAL

NEW STANDARDS

Ideal foods are healthy from start to finish: healthy seed, healthy soil, healthy growth, healthy nurturing, healthy ripening, healthy storing, and healthy consumption. That is a healthy mouthful! Ideal is the highest standard for food. It is superior to organic because it doesn't allow even the minimal toxins that even certified organic food allows. Essentially, biodynamic is what organic should be, but is not, at least on a macro scale.

I spoke to a farmer who practices sustainable biodynamic farming practices, which is about as close to ideal food as you can get. Biodynamic is a truly holistic approach to farming that takes into account ecological, social, and economically sustainable practices, according to the Biodynamic Farming and Gardening Association.[252] Research demonstrates that biodynamic, non-toxic soil preparation effectively stimulates plant growth while not harming the earth.[253] It is this perspective that provides for maximum quality, production, and benefits for both farmer and the consumer population. Biodynamic is actually ahead of organic because it allows no chemicals and works with the soil for optimal nutrition.

Continuing my conversation with this farmer on the phone, I inquired if he was going to apply for organic certification. His voice quieted as he described how he had no intention to become certified organic because the certification allows chemicals. Even if it's a small amount, he wants to do what is right and good for the earth and soil. I applaud his efforts and hope other farmers take that stance for quality over quantity food production. If more of us embark on this journey of ideal food, there will be increased availability of quality food supply.

BIODYNAMIC + AUTHENTIC ORGANIC = IDEAL

Healthnuts enjoy what is really biodynamic, or non-GMO. Healthy, real food is ideal food in that it disallows any chemicals or anything absolutely unnatural in the food production process. This just feels ideal for healthnuts. Do we need one hundred scientific research studies to tell us those GMOs or genetically engineered foods are harmful?

I've observed elderly people that grew up on an ideal food diet of a variety of different tastes and flavors. It's apparent that, with their diet, they built a proper immune foundation. We are eroding the opportunity for others to experience this level of vitality by participating in the mass production of immune-destroying foods. Those foods take many forms, but their purpose is the same: to disrupt the natural process of nutrition efficiency. Ideal is about remaining as close to the land as possible and creating products via sustainable agriculture, thereby promoting a foundation for preventive health.

SPENDING MORE

Where did we get the idea that we can spend the least amount of money on food to be healthy? What happened to the mind-set that food is an investment for lifelong health? I received an email several months ago with a scanned image of a list of the top expenditures from the early 1900s. Today, housing would lead the list for most of us. Back then, do you know what the highest expenditure was for the average household? That's right, you guessed correctly. It was food! Food was number one.[254] The mind-set has changed over the last hundred years; back then, they made food a priority. Now, we just want the most food for the least money. Whether times are good or times are hard, we need to be making our food purchases an investment in our future. The quality of food has decreased over time. Today, we spend much less on food and get minimal nutrition. Food has fallen, and housing has increased. Could this be one of the major causes of modern lifestyle diseases?

Even if we increase our food budget, usually it's for eating out. Is that healthy food? Where are those restaurants sourcing their food? From large organizations producing chemical and GMO toxic foods? Or are they accessing it from local farmers and regional sustainable growers?

You have to ask yourself, what is the true cost of saving a little on food if you end up paying more for your medical expenses? Worse, what's the cost of receiving a diagnosis of a fatal condition you could have prevented had you received the proper nutrition? Is it more important to lose weight but end up with diabetes or to eat quality foods with the side effect of weight loss, yet avoiding the debilitating diagnosis of a preventable lifelong condition?

HEALTHNUTS...

- Understand the difference between ideal foods and other natural or organic foods.
- Support initiatives that enable more ideal food production and distribution.
- Invest in ideal foods to reduce risk factors of preventable lifestyle diseases.

THE ROLE OF THE SOIL

Why is nutrition so radically different today than at any other time? Have you ever wondered how people in ancient cultures were able to live to over one hundred without disease? You would think with the better technology we have today, we would be outliving those primitive ancients. And yet, as recorded in the Bible, it is evident that some lived to hundreds of years old—even up to almost a millennium![255] Granted, they did not have the pollutants and toxins we have to deal with today. Their soils and foods were whole and not nutritionally confounded. Sure, they had some of the diseases to deal with but their food preparation processes were clean. Even ancient Jewish sanitary and dietary laws are a model foundation for healthy living and are the bedrock of our modern sanitary practices in the US.

Over the last century, a crisis has occurred in our food supply. Soil quality is not what it used to be—it has been drastically diminished in its nutritional content, especially its mineral content. You see, life and death begins with the soil. You can have the healthiest seeds in the world, but if those seeds are not cultivated on good ground, they will not take root and they will eventually die. Healthy seeds require healthy soil. Longevity is found in the soil. When soil is tarnished with unnatural chemical agents, it loses its ability to work with the seeds to maximize nutritional quality.

The focus of today's generation is on quality nutrition, but we should also be thinking about where that nutrition comes from: the soil. I don't remember hearing one lecture in elementary school about the necessity of good soil. It's almost like it was taken for granted.

We must use technology to our advantage to help replenish what is lost in the soil. But we need to do it in an ideal way that does not artificially modify the food. We need to work with the area in which we live. I firmly believe that every geographic region has the capacity to do something amazing when it comes to ideal food production. Maybe it's only a few items that are grown or cultivated, but with every healthnut working together, we can have local and regional supplies that cover the necessities of nourishing food. It's not really an option anymore. It's become a necessity for survival and for a thriving quality of life.

We've been in a painful state of lifestyle degenerative disease flux. Consider the healthcare forecast over the next twenty years.[256] Projections for care costs keep rising and rising into the trillions of dollars while quality of care is deteriorating. You must not only educate yourself about the seeds your foods come from, but the quality of the soil. On a practical level, wherever you source your food, it's best if you can actually tour the farm or talk to the farmer to learn about the soil of the foods you consume. Healthnuts know that now, more than ever, there is a desperate need for optimal nutrition and that is why they pursue fueling their bodies correctly and consistently.

HEALTHNUTS...

- Pursue the quality soil of historical times for longevity and increased quality of life.
- Avoid increased healthcare costs associated with nutritionally deprived foods.
- Use technology to cultivate real soil instead of inventing fake soils.

15

HEALTHNUT NOURISH

What if I were to walk into your house and open your pantry or fridge? What would I find? Hopefully, I would see that at a minimum, 70% of your food is whole real food and the other 30%, at a maximum, is packaged real food. Healthnuts keep their fridge and pantries stocked with healthy foods. Appetites are normal! We should not suppress a natural appetite. We should enjoy our food. It should not be a struggle or something we constantly have to avoid just to stay healthy. When you provide your body what it requires for growth and nourishment, you'll have more energy, better sleep, and more strength to work.

The following list of healthy food options will help you prioritize your food choices for a healthy lifestyle. Choose the foods you want based on the lifestyle you prefer. If you like meat, go for it. If you don't, stick with vegetarian or vegan. You have options.

As you read over the list, please keep in mind that there is a priority for which sources you choose as you purchase food. In virtually all instances, the ideal source for your food is local and biodynamic. But if this is not available, certified organic would be next best. Buying conventional real foods are a last resort.

I've organized the list into the following:

Healthnut Food Category: In this section, I describe the healthy food. I've provided the overall food categories including fruits, vegetables, seeds/nuts/oils, beans/grains, meats, fish, dairy/eggs, and sweeteners. Most important, you must consume nutrient-dense foods. Energy-dense foods are typically higher in fats and proteins. Nutrient-dense foods are lower in calories but higher in vitamins, minerals, phytochemicals, and other micronutrients.[257] Typically, fruits, vegetables, nuts, seeds, grains, and beans will have a higher nutrient density per calorie. Fish, meats, dairy, eggs, and sweeteners or baked goods will have the lowest nutrient density per calorie.

Healthnut Benefits: In this section, I provide the three main benefits to each food category.

Healthnut Reference Key: In this section, I provide the key terms for the specific food category. The key may include insulin-friendly items that are lower on the glycemic index and load. The glycemic index rates carbohydrates on their rate of conversion to glucose within the human body. However, these are just average estimates and may not apply to all food sources. For an exhaustive list of many foods and meals, check out the International Tables of Glycemic Index and Glycemic Load Values.[258] Be mindful of the glycemic index and load, especially if you need to control blood sugar and reduce foods that inhibit fat or unhealthy weight loss. Beware, just because a food is low-glycemic does not necessarily mean it's healthy!

The key will also show you which foods may be higher in pesticides, so you can purchase the biodynamic version. It will also show you which foods are lower in pesticides, in case you are on a budget or have limited food availability and are not able to purchase the biodynamic or organic versions. Finally, the key will reference foods with higher levels of beneficial compounds.

Healthnut Food Options: In this section, I provide what I believe are the most popular foods within each food category. There are absolutely many other healthful foods as well, but this will give you a starting point to recognize better-for-you foods.

Healthnut Consideration: In this section, I provide information specifically related to each list of foods. Please remember that my lists inside each category are only a starting point: certainly, there are foods in certain parts of the world that may be higher or lower in glycemic index or pesticides on this list. So make sure you always check with your local or online food suppliers to verify their standards in reference to the following guide.

Please note, if you are required to be on a special medical diet such as gluten-free or dairy-free, or if you have a preferred diet such as vegan or no sugar, just skip the foods that don't apply to you!

HEALTHNUTS...

- Identify the food categories and foods that work best for them individually.
- Prioritize healthy food options based on healthy living principles.
- Add more nutrient-dense, low-grade inflammation-reducing, and cell-protecting foods.

HEALTHNUT HYDRATION

Water is vital. You can go for days or even longer without food, but you can only last a very short time without water. Your body is mostly composed of water (55%–75%). You get most of your water from beverages and almost a quarter from food.[259] Water, herbal teas, and even herbal-infused waters are an excellent substitute for unhealthy sugar beverages and are inversely associated with OB.[260] Remember, our bodies are often water-deprived rather than food-deprived. You should make it a priority to drink your body's required amount of healthy water throughout the day. Researchers estimate that the average recommended water intake ranges from 2–3 liters per day.[261] Some experts recommend one ounce per pound of body weight. Others will recommend about one ounce per kilogram of bodyweight. Water consumption is also highly subjective and is based on a variety of factors such as weight, height, and activity level. [262]

Just as important as the amount of water that you drink, however, is the quality of the water. As much as it is possible, drink pure water without toxins or other contaminants. I know there are some health experts who promote special water, such as alkaline or ionized waters. This will not necessarily produce alkalinity within your body.[263] I would advise to verify any water claims and choose the most verifiably pure water you can find.

Ideally we would all juice and blend fresh vegetables and fruits daily for drinking—but that is too challenging and time-consuming for most of us.

Alternatively, although many store bought juices are limited in beneficial nutrients and enzymes because of high temperature pasteurization or the addition of unnecessary preservatives or additives, there is a new cold-pressed high pressure pasteurization technique (HPP) that provides some benefits of pasteurization (reducing harmful bacteria) while preserving more nutrients and enzymes.

Fermented beverages, also an option, can maximize the digestion and absorption of nutrients. If going this route, it's preferable to consume raw, unpasteurized products. As with any beverage, read the labels carefully to make sure it is reputable, unless you decide to make your own cultured drinks. Regardless of the processing, if there is a lot of sugar without fiber or there are any additives, you may have to avoid it. Even an HPP or raw unpasteurized juice without preservatives or additives may contain a high amount of sugar with or without fiber (if from real fruit with fiber it metabolizes differently). There are, of course, pros and cons to fiber versus non-fiber. Without fiber, you have smooth-tasting juice with more sugar along with the potential for blood sugar spike. With fiber, the taste is rough, the drink slows the digestive process, and your blood sugar may not be as impacted.

HYDRATION OPTIONS

+ Fermented Beverage (fresh raw/unpasteurized)
+ Flavored Water (fruit-infused)
+ Flavored Water (herbal-infused)
+ Fruit Juice (blended)
+ Fruit Juice (cold-pressed/fiber)
+ Fruit Juice (fresh, raw)
+ Herbal Teas
+ Vegetable Juice (blended)
+ Vegetable Juice (cold-pressed/fiber)
+ Vegetable Juice (fresh, raw)
+ Water (pure/contaminant-free)

HEALTHNUT KEY

1. Review processing method, whether it's raw, HPP, or purified.

2. Review sugar content per serving (the lower the better).

3. Review additives/preservatives (none is best!).

HEALTHNUT CONSIDERATIONS:[264]

- 99%–100% pure reverse osmosis water is best (contaminant-free).
- Optional to add minerals, use baking soda, or other formulas for "alkalinity."
- Optional to modify the water to have a negative oxidation-reduction potential.

HEALTHNUTS...

- Understand pure water is the most vital "nutrient" and critical for most body functions.
- Drink verifiably tested clean and pure water with absolutely no chemicals or additives.
- Avoid plastic bottled water unless traveling or in an emergency (use glass or stainless steel).

HEALTHNUT FRUITS

FRUIT BENEFITS

- Fiber supports healthy colon function.
- Antioxidants and polyphenols combat free radical damage and aging.
- High quantity of vitamins and minerals

HEALTHNUT KEY

* Lower on glycemic index[265]

! Higher in pesticides, buy organic or biodynamic.[266]

+ Higher levels of polyphenols and antioxidants [267, 268]

HEALTHNUT FRUIT OPTIONS

- Apple*+!
- Apricot*+
- Avocado*

- Banana
- Blackberry+!
- Blueberry+!

- Cantaloupe
- Cherimoya
- Cherry+!
- Clementine
- Coconut*
- Cranberry
- Currant (black or red)+
- Date
- Elderberry+
- Fig
- Goji Berry+
- Gooseberry+
- Grape+!
- Grapefruit
- Honeydew
- Huckleberry+
- Kiwi*
- Kumquat
- Lemon
- Lime
- Mango*
- Nectarine!
- Orange*
- Papaya
- Passion Fruit
- Peach*!
- Pear*!
- Pineapple
- Plum*+!
- Pluot!
- Pomegranate
- Prune+
- Raisin
- Raspberry+!
- Starfruit
- Strawberry+!
- Super fruits (Other)+
- Tangerine
- Tangelo
- Watermelon

HEALTHNUT CONSIDERATIONS

- Fruits are bursting with living flavors, colors, and cell protectors. Polyphenols are the most abundant preventive protectors.

- Whole fruits that include fiber are most useful for your body. I don't recommend juicing fruits unless it's mixed with fiber or unless you drink it alongside a meal. The purpose of limiting straight fruit juices is to limit the glycemic spike from the fruit sugars, which is typically fructose.

- However, fruit sugar from real fruits does not metabolize the same way as typical sugary beverages. I would much rather juice fruits without any additives than purchase a store-bought juice. There are a several exceptional companies with newer juice extraction technology that eliminate harmful bacteria while preserving the nutrients. These provide the beneficial nutrients and are much better than high-heat pasteurization.

+ Don't forget about other incredibly healthy by-products of fruit, such as apple cider vinegar!

+ Unfortunately, conventional and even some organic soft fruits are sprayed or contaminated with chemicals. Some examples include berries, grapes, peaches, and pears. Please note this also varies based on where the produce is sourced.

+ Fruits with thick skins, such as pineapple, oranges, and melons, contain fewer chemicals because of the protective covering. Feel free to choose non-organic if on a budget.

HEALTHNUTS...

- Eat fruits with fiber.
- Use fruits for in between meal "snacks" instead of unhealthy foods.
- Drink freshly squeezed juices in moderation.

HEALTHNUT VEGETABLES

VEGETABLE BENEFITS

+ Abundant source of fiber to support healthy elimination

+ Phytochemicals and polyphenol compounds are cell protectors.

+ High quantity of vitamins and minerals

HEALTHNUT KEY

* Higher levels of micronutrients and phytochemicals[269]

! Higher likelihood of pesticides; buy organic or biodynamic if possible.[270]

+ Higher levels of polyphenols[271]

HEALTHNUT VEGETABLE OPTIONS

- Artichoke*+
- Asparagus*+
- Beet
- Beet Greens
- Bok Choy*
- Broccoli*+
- Broccoli Sprout*+
- Brussels Sprout*
- Cabbage*
- Carrot*+!
- Cauliflower*+
- Celery*!
- Collard Green*!
- Cucumber!
- Daikon (white radish)
- Dandelion
- Eggplant
- Fermented Vegetables*
- Garlic
- Green Bean+
- Kale*!
- Kelp
- Kohlrabi*
- Kombu
- Leek
- Lettuce (Butter)!
- Lettuce (Green)*+!
- Lettuce (red leaf and romaine)*!
- Mizuna Greens
- Mushroom (brown and white)
- Mushroom (Maitake and Shitake)*
- Mustard Green*
- Nori
- Okra
- Olive+
- Onion (red, white, and yellow)+
- Parsnip
- Pea (snow and snap)
- Pepper (bell and hot)*!
- Pepper (Sweet)*+
- Potato (Sweet)!
- Potato!
- Pumpkin+
- Radish*
- Rutabaga*
- Scallion
- Shallot+
- Spinach*+!
- Squash (Acorn)*
- Squash (other)
- Super Vegetables (Other)*+

- Swiss Chard*
- Tatsoi
- Tomato (Regular)*+
- Tomato (Cherry)*+!
- Turnip*
- Turnip Greens
- Wakame
- Watercress*
- Yam
- Yarrow*
- Zucchini*
- Herb/Spice/Tea Options:
- Arugula*
- Basil*+
- Bay Leaf*
- Capers+
- Celery Seed+
- Chive*
- Cilantro*
- Cinnamon+
- Clove+
- Coriander
- Cumin+
- Curry+
- Dill*
- Endive
- Fennel
- Ginger+
- Horseradish
- Hyssop
- Lemon*+
- Mint
- Mustard
- Oregano*+
- Parsley*+
- Rosemary*+
- Peppermint*+
- Sage+
- Spearmint*+
- Star anise+
- Tea (Green)*+
- Tea (Variety)*+
- Thyme*+
- Turmeric+

HEALTHNUT CONSIDERATIONS

- Vegetables are the foundation of healthy living and provide a wide array of vitamins and minerals. Most people do not consume enough vegetables and are deficient in essential minerals and phytochemicals that protect the cells.

- It's best to get your vitamins and minerals from eating whole or drinking juiced vegetables. Juicing vegetables is one of the healthiest things you can do. Teas are another great option. Green tea, for example, is rich in antioxidants and polyphenols, which has positive effects on cholesterol, reduces the risk of heart disease, various cancers, diabetes, and digestive issues, and improves the metabolism.[272]

+ Specialty cultured or fermented vegetables and herbs include raw/vegan sauerkraut and kimchi. These provide a wide variety of nutrients such as live enzymes to digest food and immune boost, and other phytochemicals. Fermentation is one of the best methods to add beneficial bacteria to the gastrointestinal tract.

+ Most vegetables, herbs, and spices are low on the glycemic index. Exceptions include specific root vegetables such as potatoes.

+ Some of the higher chemical vegetables include celery, cucumbers, kale, lettuce, peppers, potatoes, spinach, and tomatoes. As with fruits, the vegetables' source location will determine amount of chemicals.

+ Lower chemical options include asparagus and onions. Feel free to choose non-organic if on a budget.

HEALTHNUTS...

• Drink vegetables raw or eat raw/lightly steamed in unlimited amounts (there's your main course!).

• Understand some vegetables are better assimilated raw while others are best eaten cooked.

• Use fresh and dried herbs and spices instead of other unnatural condiments in foods.

HEALTHNUT SEEDS, NUTS, AND OILS

SEED/NUT/OIL BENEFITS

+ Heart-healthy fats such as omega-3s

+ Healthy oils reduce low-grade inflammation.

+ Fat-soluble vitamins and trace minerals

HEALTHNUT KEY [273]

* Higher levels of micronutrients and phytochemicals.

! Higher likelihood of pesticides; buy organic, biodynamic, or shelled.

+ Higher levels of polyphenols.

SEED/NUT/OIL OPTIONS

- Almond+!
- Avocado Oil!
- Brazil!
- Cashew!
- Chestnut*+
- Chia Seed!*
- Coconut (oil, chips, and shreds)!
- Borage Seed (Oil)
- Filbert
- Flax Seed (brown, golden, and oil)!*
- Grape Seed (Oil)
- Hazelnut*+!
- Hemp Seed (and oil)!
- Macadamia Nut
- Macadamia (Oil)
- Nut Milks (Variety)!
- Olive (Oil)+!
- Pecan*+
- Pine Nut
- Pistachio!*
- Pumpkin Seed!*
- Pumpkin Seed (Oil)!
- Seed Milk (Variety)!
- Sesame Seed (and oil)!*
- Sunflower Seed!*
- Walnut (and oil)+*!

HEALTHNUT CONSIDERATIONS

- Does eating fat make you fat? Yes and no. Although fat calories are the densest, not all fat is created equal. Nuts, seeds, and some oils have beneficial fat burning properties. Some experts believe oils are not necessarily the healthiest choice. I include them as an option for those of you that prefer the oil. As always, use with discretion.

- Most nuts, seeds, and oils will be lower on the glycemic index.

- Nuts, seeds, and oils are best purchased organic and biodynamic. Although it is not the same as the fat in animal flesh, toxins are more easily concentrated in fats. Try to always purchase raw or extra-virgin, cold-pressed, varieties.

+ You can make your own nut and seed milks. You'll need a high-powered blender, cheesecloth, and water. You can use a light sweetener if you need to.

+ Be aware that nuts and seeds may process on machinery with other nuts, seeds, and unhealthy soy. Although manufacturers should clean the machines before a new run, you may see on packages a warning about the potential of allergic contamination.

HEALTHNUTS...

- Use caution on the overuse of oils, which may contribute to OB.
- Grind or soak nuts and seeds to make them more digestible.
- Choose nuts, seeds, and oils processed from allergy-free manufacturing facilities.

HEALTHNUT BEANS, LEGUMES, AND GRAINS

BEAN/LEGUME/GRAIN BENEFITS

+ Provide fiber to support bowel function

+ Higher vegetarian protein source

+ Contain vitamins, minerals, and other micronutrients

HEALTHNUT KEY

* Lower on glycemic index[274]

! Higher likelihood of pesticides; buy organic or biodynamic.

+ Higher levels of nutrients for beans or legumes[275, 276]

BEAN/LEGUME/GRAIN OPTIONS

+ Amaranth!

+ Beans (All)+!

+ Bean (Black)*+!

+ Bean (Garbanzo)*+!

+ Bean (Kidney)*+!

+ Bean (Lima)!

- Buckwheat!
- Einkorn!
- Emmer!
- Lentil (Green)*+!
- Lentil (Red)*+!
- Millet!
- Miso*!

- Natto*!
- Oats (No Gluten)!
- Quinoa!
- Rice (Brown)!
- Rice (Wild)!
- Sprouted grain+!
- Tempeh*!

HEALTHNUT CONSIDERATIONS

- Not everyone can eat beans. I normally only eat chickpeas, lentils, or occasionally some black beans. Soaking before cooking or blending after cooking certainly makes them more digestible.

- If you have insulin resistance or type 2 diabetes, you'll have to use extreme caution while eating grains (even gluten-free). As I mentioned previously, most of the grains are not what they used to be throughout history, especially those grains which contain gluten. The only exceptions are einkorn or emmer for those who can handle these ancient grains. Remember, they still contain gluten!

- Just because the package says gluten-free does not guarantee it is 100% free of any trace of gluten. Gluten-free oats may have a small amount of gluten, for example. If you are gluten-intolerant, you'll have to avoid grains (or foods) with any trace of gluten. You'll also want the whole form of the grain instead of the processed or refined version.

- Beans or lentils marked with lower glycemic index and load are in the raw form. It is quite possible the glycemic index and/or glycemic load may adjust based on soaking or cooking beans or grains. Use with caution.

- Purchase all beans, grains, and lentils from an organic or biodynamic source. It is suspected grains may be contaminated with arsenic, for example. The ground water used in the crop production is polluted, which gets into the plant and ends up on your plate.

- Another potential source of contamination are grains or beans processed in facilities with gluten, soy, or allergenic nuts. This provides an additional level of stress on your system.

HEALTHNUTS...

- Choose lentils, beans, and some grains for additional protein and fiber.
- Are cautious with some grains with increases in blood sugar and GI issues.
- Understand gluten-free may not mean 100% free of *all* gluten.

HEALTHNUT MEATS

MEAT BENEFITS

- High-protein source for muscle/skin/hair
- Provides beneficial fats including essential fatty acids
- Vitamins, minerals, and amino acids

HEALTHNUT MEAT OPTIONS

- Beef (Variety)
- Bison
- Buffalo
- Chicken
- Deer
- Duck
- Elk
- Lamb
- Quail
- Turkey
- Wild (Other)

HEALTHNUT CONSIDERATIONS

- Meats provide an array of vitamins that are challenging to find if on a meatless diet. On the other hand, vegetarians don't have some of the negative lifestyle health issues that are associated with higher consumptions of the wrong meats.

- If you eat meat, choose grass-fed or wild if possible. Grass-fed and grass-finished means the animals did not eat grains, which fatten up cattle. If you go wild, make sure you've checked it out to be a clean source. You don't want to consume hunted meat that is diseased!

+ It's always best to trim off as much excess fat from the meat as possible, because it's the bad, saturated variety. If you choose turkey, chicken, or red meat, always buy the leanest option. Bison and wild game tend to be exceptionally lean. However, some meat, such as lamb, may have additional fat. New Zealand-based pastured lamb provides an excellent source of carnitine for helping the body use fat for energy.

+ Use caution while consuming organ meats. Some healthnuts believe strongly in eating organ meats for the beneficial vitamins and minerals while others, such as vegetarian or vegan healthnuts, will point out the high levels of dietary cholesterol and animal fats.

+ All meats should be chemical- and hormone-free. Often, meat manufacturers will say hormones are not directly consumed by the animals, but if the animals consume food with chemicals or hormones, what does that say about the meat?

+ You should always try to choose organic or biodynamic free range. Otherwise, it is questionable whether hormones were used in the feed for natural meats. It's best if you know a local or regional supplier whom you can ask directly about their farming practices.

HEALTHNUTS...
- Choose mostly lean cuts of meat and trim off most or all fat.
- Avoid hormone, antibiotic, and chemical raised meats.
- Avoid "vegetarian" grain/soy-fed meats (animals should eat grass in most cases).

HEALTHNUT FISH

FISH BENEFITS

+ Higher protein source
+ Provides beneficial fats for cardiovascular/brain health
+ Vitamins, minerals, and essential fatty acids

FISH OPTIONS

- Anchovy
- Cod
- Flounder
- Grouper
- Haddock
- Hake
- Halibut
- Mackerel
- Mahi Mahi
- Pollack
- Rock

- Salmon (Any)
- Salmon (Sockeye)
- Sardine
- Sea Bass
- Sole
- Tilapia
- Trout (Rainbow)
- Tuna (yellow or ahi)
- Whiting
- Wild Fish
- Yellow Perch

HEALTHNUT CONSIDERATIONS

- Fish are considered one of the most nutritionally complete foods. (I think they are the perfect animal food, actually.) Fish contain key fat-soluble vitamins, minerals, and are considered low carb and high in essential fatty acids and proteins. Fish are certainly blood sugar friendly.

- Choose fish that are wild fresh or frozen without any added oil or salt, and if possible, buy only fish that have been tested for contaminants. Canned fish may be consumed on occasion, but make sure there is no added salt or oil. If you have to purchase under emergency circumstances or during travel, rinse or soak in water thoroughly before consuming to remove as much sodium as possible. Small fish such as sardines and anchovies are nutritionally dense. They contain high levels of beneficial essential omega-3 fatty acids such as DHA and EPA. These oils are anti-inflammatory, brain healthy, and fat burning. Some believe omega-3s from animals are not necessary when perfectly good sources of plant omega-3s are available. I agree that plants are extremely beneficial. However, there are thousands of studies that support the benefits of essential fats from fish.

- One major issue with fish is the toxic element contamination potential. With the rise of environmental pollution, we've seen huge increases in mercury content in some of the more toxic fish such as swordfish or some forms of tuna. Therefore, it is wise to avoid even wild fish from waters that may have extensive contamination. Purchase from a reputable source that provides tests regularly.

+ Another issue I see with fish is the additives and preservatives on labels. If you flip over the frozen fish package and see chemicals added, avoid it.

HEALTHNUTS...

- Eat healthy, clean, and toxic metal-free wild fish and avoid farm-raised fish.
- Benefit from the higher protein and essential fatty acids in fish.
- Use only wild, fresh, or frozen fish and avoid canned fish with additives.

HEALTHNUT DAIRY AND EGGS

DAIRY/EGG BENEFITS

+ Higher complete protein source
+ Higher healthy fat source
+ Source of vitamins, minerals, essential fatty acids, and probiotics

DAIRY/EGG OPTIONS

+ Cow Butter
+ Cow Milk
+ Cow Cheese
+ Cultured Dairy
+ Goat Butter
+ Goat Cheese
+ Goat Milk
+ Kefir
+ Yogurt
+ Egg
+ Egg White
+ Egg Yolk

HEALTHNUT CONSIDERATIONS

+ If possible, buy raw/unpasteurized hormone/antibiotic-free, or if that's not available, buy organic raw or minimal pasteurization, hormone/antibiotic-free.

+ There is a debate between the dairy and the non-dairy crowds. Those who are in favor of dairy describe the benefits of critical fat-soluble vitamins and key minerals lacking in most diets. Proponents point out the higher fat content is beneficial and use research studies to back their claims. Often they'll describe ancillary benefits such as probiotics for healthy flora balance in the gut. Others will describe major nutrient deficiencies that may occur unless one regularly consumes real butter or unpasteurized dairy.

+ Note, eggs are not considered to be dairy. I've grouped them with dairy because eggs are considered higher on the list of intolerant foods for some. You may be intolerant to the entire egg, to the egg whites, or to the yolks. For example, I can eat egg yolks without any problems, but in the past I've had issues with egg whites.

+ Detractors believe that dairy should be either limited or eliminated. They'll cite studies that show the damaging effects of high-fat animal diets linked with cardiovascular and other lifestyle disease. They'll promote lower fat diets and, if using dairy, will prescribe it in limited amounts. Many of my doctor colleagues would recommend eliminating dairy for patients struggling with OB.

+ Dairy is better for some if you understand how it's processed and verify that it comes from clean animals. As with other food options, your best bet is to link up with a local farmer that you trust. Check your state laws as well.

+ Fermented dairy, with its associated benefits of probiotics, enzymes, fat-soluble vitamins, and immune-boosting properties, can be very helpful for some healthnuts. Examples include yogurt, kefir, and a variety of other lacto-fermented products from different cultures. Those who are vegan or vegetarian can use fermented vegetables as an alternative to fermented dairy.

+ Real dairy is certainly better than hormone or chemical dairy. Enzymatically rich raw goat cheese is one example of a healthier option.

There's a protein in milk called casein that is actually a challenge for many people to digest properly. Goat proteins resemble human milk proteins and are much easier to assimilate.

HEALTHNUTS...

- Eat dairy and eggs if the body responds positively and otherwise avoid it completely.
- Use only real, cultured, or fermented dairy and local eggs.
- May eliminate dairy and egg whites for a season for GI repair and healing.

HEALTHNUT SWEETENERS AND BAKING GOODS

SWEETENER/ BAKING GOODS BENEFITS

- Provides better-for-you sweeteners for special occasions
- Several are lower glycemic
- Provides some key nutrients (for example, the propolis in honey)

HEALTHNUT KEY TO SWEETENERS/BAKING GOODS

* Lower on glycemic index

! Higher likelihood of adulteration; use raw or unrefined, organic and extra-virgin with minimal processing

+ Higher levels of polyphenols and antioxidants[277]

SWEETENER/BAKING GOODS OPTIONS

- Avocado Oil*!
- Cacao*+!
- Dark Chocolate*+!
- Cinnamon*
- Cocao Powder*+!

- Coconut Cream!
- Coconut Flour*!
- Coconut Nectar!
- Coconut Meat*!
- Coconut Oil*!

- Coconut Palm!
- Date
- Real Fruit
- Honey !
- Maple Syrup!
- Molasses (Unsulphered Blackstrap)*
- Nutritional Yeast

- Palmyra Palm*!
- Palm Oil*!
- Sea Salt (Pink)*
- Stevia (Liquid)*
- Stevia (Powder)*
- Tapioca Starch
- Vanilla Extract

HEALTHNUT CONSIDERATIONS

- Sweeteners and baking products are only for those occasions that call for it. I do not believe eating sweeteners and/or baking products on a regular basis is conducive to a healthy lifestyle. The only exceptions, for those that can handle it, would be cinnamon, cacao, coconut, dates, honey, and maple syrup. If you can't handle the insulin spikes, you'll have to avoid sweeteners that negatively impact your blood sugar. Palmyra palm sugar is one of the most promising new sweeteners to hit the market. It is sourced from the palmyra palm tree. Mainly found in Sri Lanka and India, the palmyra palm is considered a "tree of life" because of its rich nutritional and medicinal properties.[278] It is one of the few vegetarian sources of vitamin B12 and is considered to be approximately 3% fructose and low-glycemic.

- You may wonder why I did not select coconut sugar or nectar as low glycemic. The reason is because I've not found conclusive information. Some reports state it is low and others I've found indicate it may have a negative impact on blood sugar. It may also contain up to 40% fructose, which may contribute to OB related issues (excess fructose in any form is often a culprit in brain, gut, hormonal issues). This means it is approximately 37% more fructose than palmyra palm! Some suppliers of coconut products question the sustainability of the coconut palm sugar industry and its impact on other coconut products such as the oil, flour, or flakes. The jury is still out, but I would suggest to be cautious and if you decide to use it, to make sure to find a pure and reliable source.

- What about Stevia? One randomized trial with 106 hypertensive patients found that incorporating a special Stevia extract decreased blood pressure within 3 months.[279] What if there are reactions to Stevia in other ways that stress other body regions? Your body normally perceives a sweet taste with a natural rise in blood sugar. Your body tries to match the supposed blood sugar increase with a sweet taste. When this doesn't happen, your stress hormones become unbalanced, which taxes your adrenal glands. This creates more imbalances and makes it difficult to be free from OB. So, just because something is lower on the glycemic index doesn't mean that it's good for you.

A sweetener that is considered healthy or has some beneficial nutrients will still be broken down into the body and either end up being used for energy or stored as fat. Sugars that are higher in fructose (such as honey or coconut sugar) may tax the liver, making it more difficult to lose weight. You may have to forgo sugar sources until your body becomes balanced or you reach your desired healthy weight. Your brain is also involved and will signal to your hormone, metabolic, and digestive systems to respond to sweets accordingly. Remember, the key principle is to use moderation with all sweeteners and reduce or eliminate consumption if your goal is weight loss. You can satisfy your cravings with the right sugar substitutions without overindulging.

HEALTHNUTS...

- Use better-for-you sweeteners or baked goods for special events or occasions.
- Stick to lower-glycemic sweeteners if insulin or blood sugar imbalance is an issue.
- Understand overuse of sugar feeds low-grade inflammation and increases risk for OB.

HEALTHNUT FOOD DISCOVERY

N ow that you've reviewed the master healthnut food list, you'll need to determine which real foods work best for you. In real life, you're not always going to eat just a single food by itself; instead, you're likely to combine a variety of foods. So how do you really know which meals work best for your body? I'm going to provide two systems for discovery, one general and one more specific. The first for learning what your body loves, day in and day out, is a system I call TEST, which stands for Try, Energy, System, and Time.

TEST

1. Try

+ You must be willing to try a new healthy food.

+ Try eating a healthier food for a week and reassess.

+ Once you find a healthy food you like and works well for you, stick with it.

2. Energy

+ You can often tell if the healthy food works by your energy levels.

+ Use Boost for a quick food energy assessment (see below).

+ Avoid foods that deplete your overall energy.

3. System

+ Create your ideal health system based on your results.

- An example may be a food rotation system every four days.
- Another example may be a fruit and vegetable fast one day per week.

4. Time

- It takes time to discover the foods that will work well for you.
- Time invested in healthy eating daily provides long-lasting results.
- Document your results with specific action items each week.

I've been practicing this for about twenty years now since formally studying fitness, health, and lifestyle solutions. There is much I don't know and have yet to learn, but I'm a bit wiser after learning from my own mistakes as well as others. It is never too late to start learning!

HEALTHNUTS...

- Use TEST for discovering which action steps work best.
- Readjust to any changes throughout life to maintain a healthy weight.
- Understand that a healthy lifestyle takes time and consistency.

BOOST ASSESSMENT

I've identified a quick method of determining if a food or meal works or does not work, based on how you feel afterwards. I know this sounds super simple, but sometimes we're apt to over-complicate the simple truth: when a food is healthy (read: not overloaded with caffeine and sugar!) and makes you feel energetic and pain-free—you should make it a part of your diet!

Below is a simple tool to keep track of what works for you by noting its "boost." Boost describes whether a food energizes you or de-energizes you. You can track Boost on one food or combinations for a quick assessment. Ultimately, your goal is to consume energizing foods throughout the day, and calming and relaxing nutrients later in the day. With Boost, you will assess how you feel on three different dimensions: physical, mental, and overall.

Here's how you can implement Boost testing for a meal. First, write down the contents of your meal or snack. Then, rate your physical, mental, and overall vitality or energy at the moment of eating, twenty minutes after eating, two hours after eating, and any other pertinent observations on a scale of 1 to 10.

MEAL/SNACK: SALMON SALAD (LUNCH)			
	Physical	Mental/ Emotional	Overall
Immediate	10	9 (happy!)	10
20 minutes	10	9	9
2 hours	8	9	9
Other:	(lost energy)	(everything tasted great!)	9

If you score below 7 on any of the categories, it's a pretty good indicator that what you are doing is not optimal and your health needs some improvement. If you score above 7 but below 9, then you are doing some things pretty well but could improve. If you score a 9 or 10, then your body is most likely doing very well.

As you rate, don't forget to consider your digestive system. Are you bloated, full, and burping? If so, then you may need to rethink your food planning and rotation strategy. (Of course, keep in mind that even healthy foods in the wrong combinations, anxiety, or other digestive disturbances may cause some issues.) Ultimately, food is for energy; we eat for energy, growth, and repair. Starting to recognize a food's propensity to either energize you or deplete your energy is a great first step.

HEALTHNUTS...

- Use Boost for a quick food assessment.
- Use Boost to determine energy lows and highs.
- Use Boost to understand, over time, acceptable and unacceptable foods.

NEED IDEAS FOR MEALS WITH THESE HEALTHY INGREDIENTS?
JOIN THE HEALTHNUT COMMUNITY BY VISITING **DRHEALTHNUT.COM**
FOR DELICIOUS, *REAL FOOD*, RECIPES.

SCAN TO VISIT DRHEALTHNUT.COM

PART FIVE:
DR. HEALTHNUT ACTION

HEALTHNUT BLUEPRINT

The most critical principle you can take from this book is that to experience lifelong freedom from OB, you must integrate healthier choices into your daily routine. Crash diet promoters will tell you to lose the weight fast, but they fail to mention it's really difficult to maintain that weight loss long-term. If you really want to be healthy for the rest of your life, you must live the Healthnut Life.

You must be able to approve these lifestyle decisions and be willing to do them for the rest of your life. If you go the crash diet route, you may induce a messed-up metabolism and activate other physical ailments. Frequent crash dieting is correlated with lowering your immune system, which makes you more susceptible to disease and sickness.

What's the point of dieting if it causes you to be sicker and less healthy?

That's why most of the crash diets fail over the long term and why people look for the next fad diet every year.[280] Dieters get frustrated because they have to keep counting calories or watching food portions for energy in and energy out. This is time consuming, meticulous, and difficult to maintain! And then, beyond this frustration, they find themselves gaining the weight back and end up at an unhealthier state than before they even started.[281] There are exceptions, however. I want to emphasize that some of the diets I've covered in the book will work well because they are not really crash diets, but lifestyle programs. They just use the term diet because putting "diet" in the title sells more books.

Your only responsibility is to identify your unique wellness blueprint and the foods your body responds well to. This is not a quick fix, but I believe with diligence and patience, the Healthnut Life will work for you. This is the secret to your ideal weight. If you're already at your ideal weight but just want to eat healthier, the Healthnut Life will help guide you through the process.

HEALTHNUT LIFE PRINCIPLES

Here are a few key principles to keep in mind as you begin the Healthnut Life:[282]

- Accept your present identity: it is not your past, nor will it determine your future.

- Long-term small behavior changes improve health significantly.

- Real food promotes proper digestion, a healthy brain, and positive emotions.

HEALTHNUT LIFE BENEFITS

Healthnuts don't look at their life like a diet—they practice the behaviors that keep them at a healthy weight for life. And those behaviors have huge benefits!

- You will experience more joy in your life with healthier lifestyle choices.

- You will eat the healthy foods you are motivated to eat.

- You will naturally eat the right amount of foods.

- You won't crave bad foods.

- You will eat the foods that work best with your body.

- You will learn what works for you and what doesn't.

- You'll spend less time and money doing the wrong things.

- You won't have to worry about slipping because your body is nourished.

+ Your healthy eating will become your lifetime habit.

+ You will only develop the goals that you'll do for life.

HEALTHNUT PROTOCOL

Learning your Healthnut Protocol will take some time and patience. You might say, I don't have time! I can't wait! I need a change now! What's important is that you make the lifestyle changes that will have the most impact *first*. Here's the basic protocol:

+ Add a few healthy eating behaviors.

+ Master them until they become second nature to you.

+ Increase the number of healthy lifestyle behaviors over time.

This self-monitoring behavioral approach is shown to be highly effective in scientific studies.[283] Additional studies continue to show the benefits of integrating technology in self-management lifestyle protocols.[284] Although digital health is advancing, some of the available options may seem overwhelming. If that's the case for you, apply the Healthnut Protocol to your digital health habits, as well.

I also want to remind you that it's important to consider participating in the other side of the equation for a healthy life—physical activity. Although this book focuses exclusively on eating healthy, you are welcome to use the Healthnut Life to create your preferred physical activity plan as well.

HEALTHNUT FRAMEWORK

The Healthnut Life is a coaching framework based on the scientifically tested Motivational Interviewing (MI) for assisting you in creating your ultimate lifestyle plan. The MI approach was first identified in the 1980s as a tool for overcoming addictive behaviors.[285] Today, MI is more successful than providing traditional counseling advice because it uses a variety of strategic tools and support systems to encourage effective and long-lasting behavior change.[286] I combine MI along with other synergistic integrative coaching techniques to help you to think differently, come up with new ideas or options that you've not considered, and ultimately reach your goals.[287]

Although you can adopt the Healthnut Life for any vision, we will focus on how to eat like a healthnut. Remember, any diet you choose may provide instant results, but it's the long-term results that count. Going on and off diets without actually implementing the healthnut practices I've discussed in this book will keep you in the struggle zone, not the healthy zone!

LIFETIME PARTICIPATION

You may still be thinking, *What about portion control and calorie counting? I've been told my whole life that it's necessary!* Sure, you can count calories, monitor meal portions, and all other diet tricks if you really want. If you are motivated to do it and want to maintain that for life—go for it! But really ask yourself, are you willing to count calories or monitor your portion sizes over the long haul? Or are you subconsciously planning to "quit" once you reach your ideal weight? I would caution you to realistically consider only adding those lifestyle habits that you are willing to participate in for life.

Choose real foods that you like now *and* are willing to eat for life. Choose lifestyle activities, such as swimming, biking, and walking, that you are willing to do for life. This is a much better approach to goal-setting than a restrictive approach that is virtually impossible to maintain over the long term. You'll be happier and experience better health.

As you change your lifestyle habits, you'll find your body and mind will come into alignment with those healthy habits. You'll start to do them naturally. You'll look, feel, and be healthier.

Finally, you'll have found your lifetime solution.

HEALTHNUTS...

- Identify a unique wellness blueprint.
- Practice healthy behaviors for life.
- Understand that the healthnut framework is about freedom, not restriction.

HEALTHNUT LIFE STEPS

Step #1: Rate yourself using Healthnut Inspire

Step #2: Identify your Healthnut *Aha!*

Step #3: Choose your Healthnut Fans

STEP #1: RATE YOUR HEALTHNUT INSPIRE

Reflection	Consideration	Anticipation	Engagement	Preservation
1	2	3	4	5

(You can fill in the blanks for any health or lifestyles changes, but for now, let's focus on healthy eating habits.)

1. Reflection: I am reflecting on changing _____ but not ready.

2. Consideration: I am considering changing _____ in the future.

3. Anticipation: I am anticipating I will make _____ changes soon.

4. Engagement: I am actively engaged in _____ changes now.

5. Preservation: I am preserving my _____ changes for life.

Rate your Healthnut Inspire now regarding healthy eating habit changes on a scale of 1–5, based on which blank you fill in:

Healthnut Inspire: _____

If you review your rating from the chapter 1 example, I hope you've moved from a 1 or 2 to a 3 or 4 rating. For some of your other specific health goals, you may be at a 5. Once you decide you are willing to make a change, you are already 50% of the way toward achieving your vision.

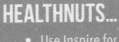

HEALTHNUTS...

- Use Inspire for targeted lifestyle activities (healthy eating, physical activity, etc.).
- Desire to reach level 5 preservation for any lifestyle activity to become "automatic."
- Understand that inspiration and self-assessment is critical to long-term lifestyle success.

STEP #2: IDENTIFY YOUR HEALTHNUT *AHA!*

1. A = Awareness
2. H = Hope
3. A = Action

Aha! is your blueprint for developing your specific roadmap for any health or lifestyle goal. This is the meat (or veggie burger, if you're vegan) of the Healthnut Life. *Aha!* gives you the accountability for your lifestyle habits. Let's begin with an example of *Aha!*

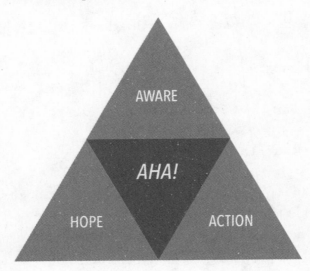

1. A = HEALTHNUT AWARENESS

Awareness starts with an understanding of the importance of your overall vision of who you want to be. This is a snapshot of you in the future. You record your future in the present as if it is happening right now. Without this big picture reminder, it's sometimes easy to lose sight in the midst of the everyday challenges you'll face. What should you keep in mind when creating your statement?

- Your awareness statement is an authentic reality for your ideal future (it's not unrealistic).

- Your awareness statement will give you a genuine stability of self-worth.

- Your awareness statement is one sentence.

- Your awareness statement is a description of your ultimate vision.

- Your awareness statement focuses on the positive aspect of your vision.

Here are some examples of awareness statements:

- I eat real food to live with vitality and be at a healthy weight.

- I eat healthy so I can be disease-free and enjoy time with family and friends.

- I make healthy food choices every day to be physically active and pain-free.

State your awareness summary statement for our healthy eating example below. Try to summarize your main motivation and ultimate vision for where you see yourself.

Your Healthnut Awareness Statement:

_____

If you prefer, go ahead and grab a sheet of paper, recorder, paintbrush, or whatever form of communication method you prefer. Be as creative as you want to be! Describe any additional details.

HEALTHNUTS...

- Develop a big picture awareness of intended lifestyle practices.
- Use present creative affirmations to confirm intention of vision.
- Abide by real-world principles to create awareness and not hype or fantasy.

2. H = HEALTHNUT HOPE

Hope is a measure of how you will take your awareness from vision to a reality. Hope is your intended target for the future that brings a measurable focus to lifestyle habits you desire. You really want these to be part of your lifestyle: don't hope for anything that is too abstract to be achieved, or too foreign to really be about "you." While awareness is broad, hope is defined and includes a measurable timeframe.

Your hope comprises the intended objectives that you are willing to commit to for life! Behavior change is often tied to your motivation, your autonomous self-regulation, and your engagement in the process.[288] As mentioned previously, if you focus your hope only on outcomes ("I want to lose weight by y") instead of on the process ("I will do x daily, no matter what"), you won't realize your hopes long term. As behavioral scientists have discovered recently, you should only choose hope goals that you are genuinely interested in and will realistically do consistently.[289]

You can have as many hopes as you like, but I would recommend starting with at least three. Keep these principles in mind when creating your hope goals:

- Choose behaviors you *want* to do, not what you *have* to do.
- Use only the tips and principles that I've discussed that feel like "you."
- Substitute unhealthy behaviors for healthier behaviors.
- Realistic: Create goals that you have control over.
- Empowering: Create goals that you are passionate about.
- Measurable: Create goals you can measure over time.
- Lasting: Create goals that can endure for life! (Although you're free to revise or change them at any time.)

Keep positive. Instead of a goal like, "In three months, I will weigh 125 pounds," which focuses on what you want to *lose*, create goals that focus on what you want to *gain*. Some examples are, "I will eat a salad for lunch every day," or "I will walk ten minutes every day," or "I will do deep breathing exercises for ten minutes every day." The positive "side effects" of these habits naturally create more success. This is not a competition, so don't measure yourself against others' success. You are only focused on what is realistic, empowering, measurable, and lasting for you.

Here are three examples of Healthnut Hopes:

+ I will eat a large salad for lunch at least 5 days per week.

+ I will always choose to purchase non-GMO foods when I eat out.

+ I will drink a glass of vegetable juice at least 5 days per week.

I want you to notice a short key phrase at the beginning of each statement. *I will. I will* is a key to unlocking your success in the Healthnut Life: it establishes commitment (only you decide), it is not optional (your direct intention), and it is powerful (your belief produces action).

Brainstorm six Healthnut Hopes:

1. _____
   _____

2. _____
   _____

3. _____
   _____

4. _____
   _____

5. _____
   _____

6. _____
   _____

In the Healthnut Life Plan, we offer space for six Healthnut Hopes—but the actual number is totally up to you! You could start with one, or start with ten. It's all about you.

HEALTHNUTS...

- Start with hopes that are lifestyle practices rather than one-time outcomes.
- Use *real* hope principles for developing realistic objectives.
- Adjust hope goals for special circumstances.

3. A = HEALTHNUT ACTION

Action is the final step in *Aha!* Action is the vehicle that drives your goals to the finish line. Take your hopes and develop your action plan weekly, daily, or hourly.

Any worthwhile healthy habit will take discipline. Starting a habit is easy, but maintaining that habit will be a lifelong challenge. The *New York Times* best seller *The Power of Habit: Why We Do What We Do in Life and Business* provides a good overview of the difficulty with achieving beneficial habits. Discipline often appears as the enemy, something both frightening and impossible.[290] As I mentioned previously, with healthier replacement habits that work for life, discipline is not drudgery, but a lifestyle.

That's an *Aha!* moment for you!

Discipline becomes second nature. What you value in life determines your commitment. If you value a healthy weight and lifestyle without preventable diseases, you will value your daily choices to realize your health goals. Instead of making a healthy lifestyle so difficult and lofty, you must break it down into bite-sized chunks.

HEALTHNUTS...

- Don't despise discipline but embrace it.
- Won't make excuses but rather invest time in health.
- Master discipline but aren't controlled by it.

Develop your action items specific to each of your six Hope goals. You'll break down each goal into a specific action item that you can use for the first week. The key to your success is commitment. There are plenty of lifestyle strategies and information tips in this book. Choose strategies that you can incorporate into your daily lifestyle. You can have as many steps as you want—they can be nutritional, active, or even spiritual! I've added some "extra" action steps beyond our food example so you can see how this may work for a more complete healthy lifestyle.

HEALTHNUT ACTION SAMPLE:

- I will eat a large salad for lunch Tuesday and Thursday (vegan version) [OR] I will eat a large chicken salad for lunch Tuesday and Thursday (meat version).

- I will only purchase non-GMO foods when I eat out on Friday.

- I will drink a large glass of vegetable juice Monday and Wednesday evening.

- I will take a brisk walk outdoors from 6-6:30 a.m. Monday, Wednesday, and Friday.

- I will stretch for 10 minutes after my walk on Monday, Wednesday, and Friday.

- I will bless my salad (vegan or non-vegan) before eating on Tuesday and Thursday.

Brainstorm six Healthnut Action Steps to accompany your six Healthnut Hopes!

I will _____
_____.

I will _____
_____.

I will _____
_____.

I will _____
_____.

I will _____
_____.

I will _____
_____.

In the Healthnut Life Plan, you'll rate yourself weekly on your success for each action, using a 1–5 scale: "1" if you made no effort to complete action, "5" if you successfully completed the action every time. Then, at the end of 7 weeks, you can average the numbers. (Note: this is why it's important to have measurable goals! You couldn't rate a goal like, "I will be more healthy.")

HEALTHNUTS...

- Integrate weekly baby action steps on a small scale toward hope goals.
- Always write action statements in positive voice of commitment ("I will").
- Design weekly action steps that are achievable at least 70% and up to 100%.

STEP #3: CHOOSE YOUR FANS

To accomplish your *Aha!* most successfully, you'll need to have support. I call this support your fans. Your fans will provide you support for your journey, encouragement for your successes, and accountability for your challenges.

Over the past ten years, I've had the privilege to coach hundreds of individuals ranging from business owners, musicians, pastors, leaders, healthcare professionals, and others that have a passion like me from all walks of life. My goal is to help them experience the life they were designed for. This is no easy task. There are many obstacles that stand between what most of us desire and what we experience. That's why we need fans.

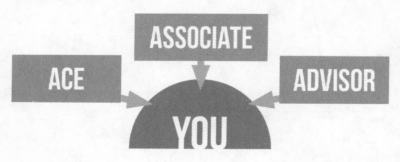

FAN BENEFITS

Fans provide many benefits that will help you to put your inspiration on cruise control. I have not met anyone who has achieved anything worthwhile in life without at least one fan. We all need fans!

- Fans will provide you excellent support.

- Fans may be close to you and can lift you up when you feel you are going to fall.

- Fans see both your good and your bad and will not desert you when things get tough.

- Fans provide encouragement.

- Fans bring out your strengths and see the best in you.

- Fans help you to most effectively align your strengths with your goals.

- Fans hold you accountable for your actions and choices.

- Fans expose blind spots or areas you may not foresee in the future.

- Fans shore up your weaknesses to overcome your biggest challenges.

FAN CATEGORIES

Research demonstrates three specific fans that are most effective for coaching people through lifestyle changes.[291] I call them your Ace, your Associate, and your Advisor. Your Ace is an expert for medical or health advice. Your Associate is your partner who's participating with you. Your Advisor is your mentor who provides additional insights.

HEALTHNUT FAN EXAMPLES:

Ace: Dr. Shannon—my expert advisor, we meet every 2 weeks.

Associate: Jane—my weekly accountability, we meet on Sundays at 2 p.m.

Advisor: Lisa—my supportive mentor, whom I can message anytime on Facebook.

Write down your three fans (or even those you hope will be your fans):

1. _____
   _____

2. _____
   _____

3. _____
   _____

What if you don't have all three available fans right now? You don't have to limit to just three or even one, but start with where you are at. Maybe your fan isn't nearby. Thanks to technology, you don't have to be limited by time or distance.

Research demonstrates remote coaching through phone and Web technology is shown to be effective.[292] A recent survey of weight-loss community participants found Internet-based support systems are convenient, encouraging, and motivational.[293] Your Adviser could be an online community, magazine, or forum! Ultimately, it's best to have at least one fan that is willing to meet with you, face-to-face or virtually, and provide support, encouragement, and accountability on a weekly basis.

What is ideal? Choose at least one Associate fan who is willing to embark on the same healthnut journey. Both of you create your *Aha!* together so that you can then become an Advisor fan to someone else. When you give to another's need, I believe you'll experience success in the goals you desire to achieve.

Once you have your fans in agreement with your *Aha!*, follow these three steps:

1. Current *Aha!*

+ Update your Associate fan with your *Aha!*

+ Include your first week's action steps.

2. Prior *Aha!*

+ Provide the results from the previous week's action steps.

3. Updated *Aha!*

◆   Provide your updated action steps for the next week.

◆   Look for patterns as you progress, and ask your Associate if they see any patterns.

◆   You may have to readjust some of these based on results.

HEALTHNUTS...

- Understand supportive fans are a must to be successful in the Healthnut Life process.
- Choose the Ace, Associate, and Advisor who are committed to long-term success.
- Use technology and other remote resources to stay on track (as needed).

HEALTHNUT LIFE PLAN

AUTOMATIC HEALTHNUT

So how do you put all of this together? Research has found that when you repeat simple behaviors and make it a pattern, you're more likely to continue doing those behaviors over time (even if you miss occasionally).[294] Your ultimate goal is do healthy behaviors until you don't have to think about them—until they become effortless.[295] We are focusing on creating healthy new behaviors, not trying to stop every bad habit. Good habits will replace bad habits if you incorporate enough good habits into your life. You won't have much time or thought for the bad habits anymore! It will take some time, so be patient and enjoy the process.

The Healthnut Life is summarized in this one statement: Do healthy actions and repeat them over time until they become automatic!

Do small changes really matter? Yes, studies demonstrate that baby-steps matter because they...

- Are easier than drastic changes.
- Are sustainable over time.
- Naturally impact body weight.
- Improve self-efficacy.
- Create more demand for healthier options.

◆ Impact every area of life (work and family).[296]

Let's review the process one more time before you get started. You'll identify your overall Healthnut Inspire. You'll develop your Healthnut Awareness statement, Healthnut Hopes, and corresponding Healthnut Action plan. Finally, you'll identify your fans and set a schedule to connect with them.

THE HEALTHNUT LIFE 7-WEEK PLAN

But what will this actually look like? Below is a sample of someone who went through the Healthnut 7-Week Life Plan, followed by a 7-Week Plan ready for you to fill out. Each week, you can update your Healthnut Life plan. You will focus on reaffirming, modifying, or replacing your hopes and action steps. You'll get better with practice.

The 7-week template is not set in stone, but is meant as a guide to help you get started. You can incorporate the Healthnut Life plan for as long as you desire or need to help you get to the place you want to be. Once you complete your first 7-week cycle, you may continue as many 7-week segments as you wish—even for life!

HEALTHNUT LIFE WEEK 1 SAMPLE

Step #1: Remember my Healthnut Inspire

Step #2: My Healthnut *Aha!*

My Healthnut Awareness Statement: _I eat healthy and live with abundant vitality so that I can enjoy a higher quality of life with friends and family._

My Healthnut Hopes and Actions (rate Actions on 1–5 scale):

Hope #1: I will _eat a large salad for lunch 5 days each week._

    Action: This week, I'll _eat a large salad for lunch on T._ [3]

Hope #2: I will _purchase non-GMO or organic healthy foods whenever I shop._

    Action: This week, I'll _purchase non-GMO foods when I shop on Sat._ [2]

Hope #3: I will _drink a large glass of vegetable juice 5 days/week._

    Action: This week, I'll _drink a large glass of vegetable juice on F._ [5]

Hope #4: I will _drink 2 liters of purified water every day._

    Action: This week, I'll _drink at least one 16 oz. glass of purified water with lemon on MWF._ [4]

Hope #5: I will _take a brisk walk outdoors for 20 minutes, 7 days per week._

    Action: This week, _I'll walk briskly from 6–6:15 a.m. on M._ [5]

Hope #6: I will _perform 15 min. of strength and flexibility exercises 3 days a week._

    Action: This week, I'll _do 5 min. of strength and flexibility on M after my walk._ [5]

> At the end of the 7 weeks, you can take the averages from each week of measuring successfully completed Healthnut Actions. If you've done everything according to plan, you should hit your goals at least 70% of the time!

Step #3: My Healthnut Fans: Week 1 Appointments:

1. Ace: _Met with Dr. Shannon to review exercise goals._

2. Associate: _Meet to review results on Su. at 2 over Skype._

3. Advisor: _Ask online community group about tips for stretching._

I'd encourage you to discuss the entire Healthnut Life with one or all of your fans before beginning. Then, share your successes for the first week and discuss your Healthnut Action steps for the next week based on your results. If you need to adjust some Action steps in week 2, wait until after an appointment with your fan.

Healthnut Score Week 1: _24 / 6 = 4_

For your Healthnut Score, combine the numbers in each box from your actions which you rated on a 1–5 scale: "1" if you made no effort to complete the action and "5" if you successfully completed the action every time. Then, divide by the number of actions for an average.

HEALTHNUT LIFE WEEK 1

Step #1: Remember my Healthnut Inspire (see page 203)
Step #2: My Healthnut *Aha!* (see page 205)

My Healthnut Awareness Statement:

_____

_____

_____.

My Healthnut Hopes and Actions (rate Actions on 1–5 scale):

Hope #1: I will _____

_____.

    Action: This week, I'll _____

_____.[   ]

Hope #2: I will _____

_____.

    Action: This week, I'll _____

_____.[   ]

Hope #3: I will _____

_____.

    Action: This week, I'll _____

_____.[   ]

Hope #4: I will _____

_____.

    Action: This week, I'll _____

_____.[   ]

Hᴏᴘᴇ #5: I will _____

_____ .

    Action: This week, I'll _____

_____ .[   ]

Hᴏᴘᴇ #6: I will _____

_____ .

    Action: This week, I'll _____

_____ .[   ]

Step #3: My Healthnut Fans: Week 1 Appointments

1. _____

_____

2. _____

_____

3. _____

_____

Healthnut Score Week 1: _____

HEALTHNUT LIFE WEEK 2 SAMPLE

Step #1: Remember my Healthnut Inspire

Step #2: My Healthnut *Aha!*

My Healthnut Awareness: *I eat healthy and live with abundant vitality so that I can enjoy a higher quality of life with friends and family.*

My Healthnut Hopes and Actions (Week 2 updates, rate Actions on 1–5 scale):

HOPE #1: I will *eat a large salad for lunch 5 days each week.*

    Action: This week, I'll *eat a large salad for lunch T and Th.* [4]

HOPE #2: I will *purchase non-GMO or organic healthy foods when I shop every week.*

    Action: This week, I'll *buy non-GMO foods at the store and local vegetables at the local farmers market on Sat.* [2]

HOPE #3: I will *drink a large glass of vegetable juice 5 days per week.*

    Action: This week, I'll *drink a large glass of vegetable juice (with a touch of lemon) M and F.* [5]

HOPE #4: I will *drink at least 2 liters of purified water every day.*

    Action: This week, I'll *drink at least 1 16 oz. glass of purified water with lemon right after I wake up M-F.* [4]

HOPE #5: I will *take a brisk walk outdoors for 20 min. 7 days per week.*

    Action: This week, I'll *walk briskly from 6–6:10 a.m. M and W.* [5]

HOPE #6: I will *perform 15 min. of strength and flexibility exercises 3 days each week.*

    Action: This week, I'll *perform 5 min. of strength and flexibility exercises on M and W after my walk.* [5]

After completing the week 2 forms, you should have a better idea whether you over- or under-committed during the first week. This is the perfect time to make adjustments. You're learning to make commitments for healthy activities. If you need to adjust your time, that's okay. You'll also want to assess how your fans are working out for you—even if you've only been in touch with one or two. They'll help you identify some critical areas or even something unexpected that you didn't notice.

Step #3: My Healthnut Fans: Week 2 Appointments

1. Ace: <u>*No meetings this week.*</u>

2. Associate: <u>*Meet with my accountability partner on Skype to review results Sun.*</u>
<u>*at 2.*</u>

3. Advisor: <u>*Inquire with community about easiest methods to juice.*</u>

> I always like to use the same time schedule for simplicity purposes–but choose what works best for you! Your other fans, Ace and Advisor, may only be available at certain times, so you may have to provide summaries of progress and be flexible.

HEALTHNUT CONSIDERATIONS

- How well are your time commitments working for you? *I'm feeling good right now because I'm taking this in small steps. Instead of grabbing the sugary beverage, I'm drinking a glass of fresh juice. I feel the energy and difference in my body.*

- How has your fan feedback been for you? *Susan, my associate accountability partner, has been wonderful. We have similar values so it's pretty easy to help each other.*

- Were there any surprises this week? *The juicing takes a lot of time! It's not so much the actual juicing but the preparation and cleanup. I'm asking the community what they've found to be helpful in juicing this week.*

Healthnut Score Week 2: <u>25 / 6 = 4.17</u>

HEALTHNUT LIFE WEEK 2

Step #1: Remember My Healthnut Inspire (see page 203)

Step #2: My Healthnut *Aha!* (see page 205)

My Healthnut Awareness:

_____

_____

_____

My Healthnut Hopes and Actions (Week 2 updates, rate Actions on 1–5 scale):

HOPE #1: I will _____

_____.

    Action: This week, I'll _____

_____.[   ]

HOPE #2: I will _____

_____.

    Action: This week, I'll _____

_____.[   ]

HOPE #3: I will _____

_____.

    Action: This week, I'll _____

_____.[   ]

HOPE #4: I will _____

_____.

    Action: This week, I'll _____

_____.[   ]

Hope #5: I will _____

_____.

    Action: This week, I'll _____

_____.[ ]

Hope #6: I will _____

_____.

    Action: This week, I'll _____

_____.[ ]

Step #3: My Healthnut Fans: Week 2 Appointments

1. _____

_____

2. _____

_____

3. _____

_____

HEALTHNUT CONSIDERATIONS

- How well are your time commitments working for you?
- How has your fan feedback been for you?
- Were there any surprises this week?

Healthnut Week 2 Score: _____

HEALTHNUT LIFE WEEK 3 SAMPLE

Once you've made it to week 3, you're well on your way to establishing new habits. The first two weeks are always the most challenging. Look at your biggest challenge and the easiest step and evaluate whether to scale back or step up.

Step #1: Remember my Healthnut Inspire

Step #2: My Healthnut *Aha!*

My Healthnut Awareness: *I eat healthy and live with abundant vitality so that I can enjoy a higher quality of life with friends and family.*

You may feel like you are repeating yourself every week, but there is a purpose. You are cementing in your mind, through your actions, on a weekly basis, the importance of your inspiration, awareness, hopes, and actions.

My Healthnut Hopes and Actions (Week 3 updates; rate Actions on 1–5 scale):

HOPE #1: I will *eat a large salad for lunch 5 days each week.*

    Action: This week, I'll *eat a large salad for lunch M, W, and Th.* [3]

HOPE #2: I will *purchase non-GMO or organic healthy foods when I shop every week.*

    Action: This week, I'll *buy non-GMO foods at the store and local fruits and vegetables at the farmers market on Sat.* [3]

HOPE #3: I will *drink a large glass of vegetable juice 5 days per week.*

    Action: This week, I'll *drink a large glass of vegetable juice (with a touch of lemon) MWF.* [5]

HOPE #4: I will *drink 2 liters of purified water every day.*

    Action: This week, I'll *drink at least 1 16 oz. glass of purified water with lemon every morning 30 min. before I eat.* [3]

HOPE #5: I will *take a brisk walk outdoors for 20 min., 7 days per week.*

    Action: This week, I'll *walk briskly from 6–6:10 a.m. MWF.* [4]

Hᴏᴘᴇ #6: I will *stretch for 10 min., 7 days per week after each walk, while deep breathing for at least 5 min.*

Action: This week, I'll *stretch for 5 min. after my walks MWF, and practice deep breathing during the stretch time for at least 2 min.* [4]

Step #3: My Healthnut Fans: Week 3 Appointments

1. Ace: *No meetings this week.*

2. Associate: *Meet with my accountability partner on Skype to review results Sun. at 2.*

3. Advisor: *Share updates with community online of what's working well and ask about emergencies.*

HEALTHNUT CONSIDERATIONS:

- **What went well this week?**
  Bob from the online community had a great suggestion. He's got a busy schedule like me and said I could do the juicing in one day for the whole week. I could use a vacuum sealer and mason jars to remove the air out of the juice and store in the refrigerator. Love the idea!

- **What's your biggest challenge?**
  This was a very challenging week. I had an unexpected family emergency on W and missed one of my physical activity days. I really noticed the difference.

- **How do you feel overall?**
  My sleep was not as good and I wasn't as energized on W.

Healthnut Week 3 Score: *22 / 6 = 3.67*

Don't forget to create Hopes and Actions that are measurable!

HEALTHNUT LIFE WEEK 3

Step #1: Remember my Healthnut Inspire (see page 203)

Step #2: My Healthnut *Aha!* (see page 205)

My Healthnut Awareness:

_____

_____

_____

My Healthnut Hopes and Actions (Week 3 updates; rate Actions on 1–5 scale):

HOPE #1: I will _____

_____.

    Action: This week, I'll _____

_____.[   ]

HOPE #2: I will _____

_____.

    Action: This week, I'll _____

_____.[   ]

HOPE #3: I will _____

_____.

    Action: This week, I'll _____

_____.[   ]

HOPE #4: I will _____

_____.

    Action: This week, I'll _____

_____.[   ]

HOPE #5: I will _____

_____.

   Action: This week, I'll _____

_____.[ ]

HOPE #6: I will _____

_____.

   Action: This week, I'll _____

_____.[ ]

Step #3: My Healthnut Fans: Week 3 Appointments

1. _____

_____

2. _____

_____

3. _____

_____

HEALTHNUT CONSIDERATIONS:

- What went well this week?
- What's your biggest challenge?
- How do you feel overall?

Healthnut Week 3 Score: _____

HEALTHNUT LIFE WEEK 4 SAMPLE

Step #1: Remember my Healthnut Inspire

Step #2: My Healthnut *Aha!*

My Healthnut Awareness: *I eat healthy and live with abundant vitality so that I can enjoy a higher quality of life with friends and family.*

My Healthnut Hopes and Actions (Week 4 updates; rate Actions on 1–5 scale):

HOPE #1: I will *eat a large salad for lunch 5 days each week.*

    Action: This week, I'll *eat a large salad for lunch M, T, W, and Th.* [5]

HOPE #2: I will *purchase non-GMO or organic healthy foods when I shop every week.*

    Action: This week, I'll *buy non-GMO and organic frozen foods at the store and local organic fruits and vegetables at the farmers market on Sa.* [3]

HOPE #3: I will *drink a large glass of vegetable juice 5 days per week.*

    Action: This week, I'll *drink a large glass of vegetable juice M, T, W, & F.* [4]

HOPE #4: I will *drink 2 liters of purified water every day.*

    Action: This week, I'll *drink at least one 16 oz. glass of purified water after I awake every day. I'll also drink 16 oz. of water 30 min. prior to lunch.* [4]

HOPE #5: I will *take a brisk walk outdoors for 20 min., 7 days per week.*

    Action: This week, I'll *walk briskly from 6–6:15 a.m. M–F.* [5]

HOPE #6: I will *stretch for 10 min., 7 days per week after each walk. I will also incorporate deep breathing into my stretch time for at least 3 min.*

    Action: This week, I'll *stretch for 5 min. after my walks M–F and practice deep breathing during the stretch time for at least 2 min.* [4]

Step #3: My Healthnut Fans: Week 4 Appointments

1. Ace: *No meetings this week.*

2. Associate: *Meet with my accountability partner on Skype to review results Sun. at 2.*

3. Advisor: *Share updates with community online about what's working well.*

HEALTHNUT CONSIDERATIONS:

- **What inspires you most about your new lifestyle?** *I'm happy to have a plan for my lifestyle–before it was just hit or miss. I would try something and it would fizzle. Now, I have everything I need to continue this lifestyle.*

- **What would you like to improve?** *I've found I'm pretty sore after strength training. Not sure if this goes away. Maybe I need to ask Dr. Shannon about that?*

- **How well do your actions align with your hopes?** *I feel like this combination is what I want to do. No one is telling me what hopes or action steps to do. I get to be the boss of my wellbeing and I like it that way.*

At the end of week 4, you are almost 30 days into the Healthnut Life. You may feel like you're doing great. Or, you may feel like you've hit some challenges. Obstacles happen in life. Use your fans (especially your Associate fan) as a resource to help you overcome difficulties. Consider what inspires you most about this process. Think about how you can improve. The solutions are inside of you.

Healthnut Week 4 Score: _25 / 6 = 4.17_

HEALTHNUT LIFE WEEK 4

Step #1: Remember my Healthnut Inspire (see page 203)

Step #2: My Healthnut *Aha!* (see page 205)

My Healthnut Awareness:

_____

_____

_____

My Healthnut Hopes and Actions (Week 4 updates; rate Actions on 1–5 scale):

Hope #1: I will _____

_____.

    Action: This week, I'll _____

_____.[ ]

Hope #2: I will _____

_____.

    Action: This week, I'll _____

_____.[ ]

Hope #3: I will _____

_____.

    Action: This week, I'll _____

_____.[ ]

Hope #4: I will _____

_____.

    Action: This week, I'll _____

_____.[ ]

HOPE #5: I will _____

_____.

    Action: This week, I'll _____

_____.[   ]

HOPE #6: I will _____

_____.

    Action: This week, I'll _____

_____.[   ]

Step #3: My Healthnut Fans: Week 4 Appointments

1. _____

_____

2. _____

_____

3. _____

_____

HEALTHNUT CONSIDERATIONS:

- What inspires you most about your new lifestyle?
- What would you like to improve?
- How well do your actions align with your hopes?

Healthnut Week 4 Score: _____

HEALTHNUT LIFE WEEK 5 SAMPLE

> Before filling in Week 5, step back and reconsider the process. Don't just think about the challenge as something mechanistic. You can certainly exercise your creativity. You may feel like you want to keep track in a different way. Go for it! Do whatever works best for you. Consider which lifestyle actions you either never knew about, or were always there, but you just didn't have the motivation to do until now.

Step #1: Remember my Healthnut Inspire

Step #2: My Healthnut *Aha!*

My Healthnut Awareness: *I eat healthy and live with abundant vitality so that I can enjoy a higher quality of life with friends and family.*

My Healthnut Hopes and Actions (Week 5 updates; rate Actions on 1–5 scale):

HOPE #1: I will *eat a large salad for lunch 5 days each week.*

    Action: This week, I'll *eat a large salad for lunch M, T, W, Th, and F.* [4]

HOPE #2: I will *purchase non-GMO or organic healthy foods when I shop every week.*

    Action: This week, I'll *buy non-GMO and organic foods at the store and lo-cal organic fruits and vegetables at the farmers market on Sat.* [5]

HOPE #3: I will *drink a large glass of vegetable juice 5 days per week.*

    Action: This week, I'll *drink a large glass of vegetable juice M–F.* [4]

HOPE #4: I will *drink 2 liters of purified water every day.*

    Action: This week, I'll *drink at least a 16 oz. glass of purified water right after I wake, another 30 min. prior to lunch, and another after my walk M–F.* [4]

HOPE #5: I will *take a brisk walk outdoors for 20 min. 7 days per week.*

    Action: This week, I'll *walk briskly from 6–6:15 a.m. M–F. I'll walk briskly from 8–8:10 a.m. Sat. and Sun.* [4]

HOPE #6: I will *stretch for 10 min., 7 days per week after each walk. I will also incorporate deep breathing into my stretch time for at least 3 min.*

    Action: *This week, I'll stretch for 5 min. after my walks M–Su. and practice deep breathing during the stretch time for at least 2 min.* [5]

Step #3: My Healthnut Fans: Week 5 appointments with my fans

1. Ace: *Meet with Dr. Shannon to discuss muscle soreness.*

2. Associate: *Meet with my accountability partner on Skype to review results Sun. at 2.*

3. Advisor: *Ask community about their experience with muscle soreness.*

HEALTHNUT CONSIDERATIONS:

- What have you learned most this week? *I learned lifestyle is a choice. I am making the right choices now. I am living it and seeing the results.*

- What have your fans taught you? *Dr. Shannon told me that some soreness is normal. There's a difference between acute pain and general soreness. I mentioned that the soreness goes away after a day and it's not sharp pain–which means it's general. The community said the same thing.*

- Which lifestyle actions do you love? *I feel such a difference eating real foods. I am more energized which gives me the pep I need to exercise regularly.*

Healthnut Week 5 Score: _26 / 6 = 4.33_

HEALTHNUT LIFE WEEK 5

Step #1: Remember my Healthnut Inspire (see page 203)

Step #2: My Healthnut *Aha!* (see page 205)

My Healthnut Awareness:

_____

_____

_____

My Healthnut Hopes and Actions (Week 5 updates; rate Actions on 1–5 scale):

HOPE #1: I will _____

_____.

   Action: This week, I'll _____

_____.[ ]

HOPE #2: I will _____

_____.

   Action: This week, I'll _____

_____.[ ]

HOPE #3: I will _____

_____.

   Action: This week, I'll _____

_____.[ ]

HOPE #4: I will _____

_____.

   Action: This week, I'll _____

_____.[ ]

Hope #5: I will _____

_____.

    Action: This week, I'll _____

_____.[ ]

Hope #6: I will _____

_____.

    Action: This week, I'll _____

_____.[ ]

Step #3: My Healthnut Fans: Week 5 Appointments

1. _____

_____

2. _____

_____

3. _____

_____

HEALTHNUT CONSIDERATIONS:

- What have you learned most this week?
- What have your fans taught you?
- Which lifestyle actions do you love?

Healthnut Week 5 Score: _____

HEALTHNUT LIFE WEEK 6 SAMPLE

Step #1: Remember my Healthnut Inspire

Step #2: My Healthnut *Aha!*

My Healthnut Awareness: <u>*I eat healthy and live with abundant vitality so that I can enjoy a higher quality of life with friends and family.*</u>

> As you get close to the end of this first 7-week phase, which hopes are you finding are not yet automatic? Which do you have to keep looking at your schedule to be reminded of?

My Healthnut Hopes and Actions (Week 6 updates; rate Actions on 1–5 scale):

HOPE #1: I will <u>*eat a large salad for lunch 5 days each week.*</u>

Action: This week, I'll <u>*eat a large salad for lunch M–F. I'm on vacation so I'm going to be make the best choice to add only healthy salad toppings like avocado.*</u>   [4]

HOPE #2: I will <u>*purchase non-GMO or organic healthy foods when I shop every week.*</u>

Action: This week, I'll <u>*choose the healthiest non-GMO foods when I eat out. I'll also stop by the store before leaving to select some health "real food" snacks that will keep my blood sugar in check and my stomach satisfied.*</u>   [4]

HOPE #3: I will <u>*drink a large glass of vegetable juice 5 days per week.*</u>

Action: This week, I'll <u>*locate a store where I can purchase a healthy pre-made vegetable juice or a cafe that serves fresh juices on the go.*</u>   [5]

HOPE #4: I will <u>*drink 2 liters of purified water every day.*</u>

Action: This week, I'll <u>*drink at least 4 16 oz. glasses of water throughout the day, when I can.*</u>   [4]

HOPE #5: I will <u>*take a brisk walk outdoors for 20 min., 7 days per week.*</u>

Action: This week, I'll <u>*do some physical activity for at least 15 min. each day whether a walk, swim, or bike ride.*</u>   [4]

HOPE #6: I will <u>*stretch for 10 min., 7 days per week after each walk and incorporate deep breathing into my stretch time for at least 3 min.*</u>

Action: This week, I'll *stretch for 5 min. after walking, swimming, or biking.* _____[4]

Step #3: My Healthnut Fans: Week 6 Appointments

1. Ace: *No meetings this week.* _____

2. Associate: *Meet with my accountability partner on Skype to review results F at 5.* _____

3. Advisor: *I am traveling this week for vacation so I really need some good advice from my supportive fans.* _____

HEALTHNUT CONSIDERATIONS:

- Which hopes are not "automatic" yet? *I'm doing my best to get the water and physical activity into my lifestyle. It's one thing to do this at home. It's another to do it while on vacation!*

- Which hopes are "automatic" for you? *I can choose to eat a salad and buy healthier food choices when I shop. This is in my control and comes easily.*

- Who else can you share your positive results with this week? *I've called my mom and told her about the great results I'm experiencing. She is excited to try the lifestyle plan too. I know she's at a different stage in her life and her hopes and action steps will look different from mine.*

Healthnut Week 6 Score: *25 / 6 = 4.17* _____

HEALTHNUT LIFE WEEK 6

Step #1: Remember my Healthnut Inspire (see page 203)

Step #2: My Healthnut *Aha!* (see page 205)

My Healthnut Awareness:

_____

_____

_____

My Healthnut Hopes and Actions (Week 6 updates; rate Actions on 1–5 scale):

Hope #1: I will _____

_____.

    Action: This week, I'll _____

_____.[   ]

Hope #2: I will _____

_____.

    Action: This week, I'll _____

_____ [   ]

Hope #3: I will _____

_____.

    Action: This week, I'll _____

_____ [   ]

Hope #4: I will _____

_____.

    Action: This week, I'll _____

_____ [   ]

Hope #5: I will _____

_____.

   Action: This week, I'll _____

_____ [   ]

Hope #6: I will _____

_____.

   Action: This week, I'll _____

_____ [   ]

Step #3: My Healthnut Fans: Week 6 Appointments

1. _____

_____

2. _____

_____

3. _____

_____

HEALTHNUT CONSIDERATIONS:

- Which hopes are not "automatic" yet?
- Which hopes are "automatic" for you?
- Who else can you share your positive results with this week?

Healthnut Week 6 Score: _____

HEALTHNUT LIFE WEEK 7 SAMPLE

Step #1: Remember my Healthnut Inspire

Step #2: My Healthnut *Aha!*

My Healthnut Awareness: *I eat healthy and live with abundant vitality so that I can enjoy a higher quality of life with friends and family.*

My Healthnut Hopes and Actions (Week 7 updates; rate Actions on 1–5 scale):

Hope #1: I will *eat a large salad for lunch 5 days each week.*

    Action: This week, I'll *eat a large salad for lunch M–F.* [5]

Hope #2: I will *purchase non-GMO or organic healthy foods when I shop every week.*

    Action: This week, I'll *buy non-GMO and organic foods at the store and local organic fruits and vegetables at the farmers market on Sa.* [5]

Hope #3: I will *drink a large glass of vegetable juice 5 days per week.*

    Action: This week, I'll *drink a large glass of vegetable juice (with a touch of lemon and ginger) M–F.* [4]

Hope #4: I will *drink 2 liters of purified water every day.*

    Action: This week, I'll *drink four 16 oz. glasses of water throughout the day. Three will be 30 minutes prior to my meals and the last, after my workouts.* [5]

Hope #5: I will *take a brisk walk outdoors for 20 min., 7 days per week.*

    Action: This week, I'll *walk briskly from 6–6:20 a.m. M–F and 8–8:20 a.m. Sat. & Sun.* [5]

Hope #6: I will *stretch for 10 min., 7 days per week after each walk. I will also incorporate deep breathing into my stretch time for at least 3 min.*

    Action: This week, I'll *stretch for 10 min. after my walks M–Sun. and practice deep breathing during the stretch time for at least 3 min.* [5]

Step #3: My Healthnut Fans: Week 7 appointments with my fans

1. Ace: *Doing a physical checkup with Dr. Shannon.*

2. Associate: *Meet with my accountability partner on Skype to review results Sun. at 2.*

3. Advisor: *Posting my results to the community this week.*

HEALTHNUT CONSIDERATIONS:

- How will you apply the Healthnut Life to other areas of your life? *I'm pretty confident now–I thought about applying this to decluttering my house and maybe to cooking better for my family, too–not just myself!*

- What have your family or friends noticed different about you? *My family sees me smiling more. I feel better. I'm not as stressed. Oh, and the best part, my doctor told me that I've lost 10 lbs and 4 inches!*

- How will you continue your new lifestyle? *I will continue this lifestyle. I have the inspiration, hope, and encouragement. My family is getting involved too. I hope to help others believe they can get healthier and make it automatic.*

Healthnut Week 7 Score: <u>29 / 6 = 4.83</u>

Congratulations! You completed 7 weeks of the Healthnut Life. Granted, you may have accomplished this goal your own way, which is perfectly fine. Whether you've used my system or adopted your own, what matters most is that you've learned what works well for you and what doesn't! You've discovered some insights about yourself you didn't know and some you may have forgotten about. People around you notice the difference in your attitude and aptitude. You have practiced the system that can help you pursue any lifestyle action plan you desire. Don't stop here! Continue on! Develop new lifestyle goals or keep refining the goals you've been working on.

HEALTHNUT LIFE WEEK 7

Step #1: Remember my Healthnut Inspire (see page 203)
Step #2: My Healthnut *Aha!* (see page 205)

My Healthnut Awareness:

_____

_____

_____

My Healthnut Hopes and Actions (Week 7 updates; rate Actions on 1–5 scale):

Hope #1: I will _____

_____.

   Action: This week, I'll _____

_____.[ ]

Hope #2: I will _____

_____.

   Action: This week, I'll _____

_____.[ ]

Hope #3: I will _____

_____.

   Action: This week, I'll _____

_____.[ ]

Hope #4: I will _____

_____.

   Action: This week, I'll _____

_____.[ ]

HOPE #5: I will _____

_____.

    Action: This week, I'll _____

_____.[   ]

HOPE #6: I will _____

_____.

    Action: This week, I'll _____

_____.[   ]

Step #3: My Healthnut Fans: Week 7 Appointments

1. _____

_____

2. _____

_____

3. _____

_____

HEALTHNUT CONSIDERATIONS:

- How will you apply the Healthnut Life to other areas of your life?
- What have your family or friends noticed different about you?
- How will you continue your new lifestyle?

Healthnut Score Week 7: _____

OVERALL HEALTHNUT SCORE

If desired, you now have the option to discover your overall Healthnut Score! Add up your averages from each week, and then average them, for a total Healthnut Score. Or, add up the numbers for each Hope (and its corresponding Actions) and average them for an overall Healthnut Score for the individual Hope!

You now have a record of what you've been able to accomplish for over 40 days! For the hopes and actions that you found reoccurring every week and that you successfully realized or completed, remember that it's likely you'll be able to do them for the rest of your life!

You can start the cycle over again with a new awareness, hopes, and action steps at any time. That's the beauty of the Healthnut Life. The Healthnut Life can work forever!

HEALTHNUT SYNERGY

SHARING HEALTH: IT'S ABOUT OTHERS

Healthnuts eat not just for self, but also for others. We are not on this earth just to please ourselves. When you eat healthy, you ensure your intended life expectancy. There is no reason to die from a lifestyle-provoked, preventable disease and miss quality years with your family. Whether you have a spouse, children, or grandchildren you can eat healthy for them. You'll also be a model for your family. It's evident that children follow after their parents' eating patterns. Whether you're single, married, young, old, it doesn't matter. Eating healthy is for everyone.

THE ULTIMATE GOAL

Healthnuts eat healthy to have the energy to help others fulfill their dreams. If we are living unhealthily, it is much more difficult to serve others! Just think about when you are sick—do you feel like helping someone else? No, you want to *be* helped! I'm not talking about those who struggle with a birth defect, a genetic condition, or an unplanned tragedy. Those in such situations should of course never feel that they are a burden. Rather, I'm addressing people like myself, in my twenties—so consumed with looking good and eating whatever I wanted, that I did damage to my own body and, logically, did damage to anyone else I could have helped instead of focusing on myself.

If we are well and take the preventive steps to stay well, we have the fortitude to help those less fortunate. I believe you are that influencer and are paving your path toward genuine wholeness. Being OB-free for life may be wonderful, but wholeness in every area of your life is even more ideal.

HEALTHNUTS...

- Eat healthy to get well, restore hope, and be alive!
- Eat healthy to be around for family and friends.
- Eat healthy to serve others.

HEALTHNUT SYNERGY

Healthnut Synergy is not about perfection. Take action *now*. Determine to get better today. Add one thing to your life that is healthy. I believe God has wonderful plans in store for you. He wants you to be well so you can impact our world for good. I believe that by eating healthier, you'll have more vitality to fulfill your destiny. In closing, my prayer is that you would prosper in all things and be in health, even as your soul prospers.[297]

DR. HEALTHNUT SAYS...

CONGRATULATIONS!

JOIN OUR EXCITING HEALTHNUT COMMUNITY WHERE YOU WILL BE MOTIVATED, ENCOURAGED, AND INSPIRED TO LIVE THE HEALTHNUT LIFE AT **DRHEALTHNUT.COM**.

FOR MORE INFORMATION ABOUT DR. HEALTHNUT PRODUCTS AND SERVICES OR TO SHARE YOUR RESULTS, PLEASE VISIT **DRHEALTHNUT.COM**.

SCAN TO VISIT DRHEALTHNUT.COM

NEED A HARD COPY OF THE 7-WEEK PLAN?
JOIN THE HEALTHNUT COMMUNITY BY VISITING **DRHEALTHNUT.COM**
TO DOWNLOAD A PRINTABLE VERSION OF THE 7-WEEK PLAN, AS WELL AS BONUS WEEKS!

SCAN TO VISIT DRHEALTHNUT.COM

ACKNOWLEDGMENTS

I acknowledge my heavenly Father for leading and guiding me in my passion and pursuit for wholeness. I have discovered through His wisdom that ultimate health and life comes from the Lord. I honor Him today and pray that you will experience the life-giving principles that He has revealed to me. I would like to honor my wonderful family: my lovely wife and my mother and father. Special thanks goes to Shannon Moffit for the cover photo. I would like to thank my friends, mentors, and colleagues who have inspired and encouraged me along this journey of life with their incomparable insights, dedication, and support. The best is yet to come.

APPENDIX

TESTIMONIES

"I've been reducing portions and limiting fatty and high-calorie foods and drinks on my Healthnut Life Plan. Just making this small adjustment, I've lost 10 lb. in 3 weeks! Now starting to add some simple lifestyle adjustments to keep up the momentum, such as taking stairs instead of the elevator at the office. I'm sleeping better and feeling great with just a few simple changes in just one week!"

—*Drew*
Phoenix, AZ

"I'm fired up and loving this! Dr. Healthnut has been so inspiring! I have been eating more organic/non-GMO real foods since starting with this group. This is week 3 and my fibromyalgia already feels 30–50% better with less body aches and brain fog! I had a serious junk food and sugar addiction, and am overcoming this habit by intentionally using the tools that David so graciously has given us. It gives us the power to make healthy choices and have fun while doing it! We're renewing our minds, which leads to a healthy spirit, soul and body. (Romans 12:1.)"

—*Beth*
Dallas, TX

"This book is dynamic! Other diets are boring because it's the same food all the time. You do have to enjoy eating healthy. Feeling really blessed! Since I have been making changes to my diet I have seen my daily blood sugar levels drop by an average of 20 points every time I test my sugar levels compared to the average prior to making changes in my diet. As for losing weight, I know I have lost weight because my pants and shorts are getting very loose to the point that I am starting to feel that I need to purchase a smaller waist size!"

—*Ron*
Nashville, TN

"*Diet Diagnosis* is a treasure map to better health with nuggets on every page. I love Dr. Nico's writing style because it's clear, forthright, and packed with great information to help us make our own choices about how best to improve our health. I have lost 8-plus pounds since beginning with Dr. David; I'm walking consistently and setting goals for myself that I am sticking to. I have more energy and determination to succeed. I know this is a permanent lifestyle change for me that will reap great benefits!"

—*Patricia*
Florida

"I am very much more aware of how exercise is vital for me as I am sitting most of the work day. I have been exercising at the gym a minimum of three times a week. The awareness of what Dr. Healthnut has brought to me has created so many positive changes in my diet. I'm now feeling and seeing a difference in a short amount of time! I am honored to highly recommend him. I say this with over twelve years of having coaches, mentors, and counselors who have given me wise council along the way. They were incredible coaches and leaders—and then I met David Nico. He's *gold*!"

—*Dr. Becky*
Phoenix, AZ

"I didn't know what I didn't know! That's what I discovered participating in the Healthnut Life Challenge with David Nico (Dr. Healthnut). I have been inspired by the Healthnut Life in so many ways. It is a significant tool to organize my thoughts about my hopes, ideas, support, and action steps to live in a true state of health. It is simple to create the plan by filling in the blanks. I am now cooking more, moving more, planning more, and choosing more as I now am mindful of all aspects of my health I need for health—body and soul. I recognize that it was the 'support' ingredient that was missing from my efforts. The weekly Healthnut Life Challenge coaching calls were invaluable as I gained more information every week. It was encouraging to hear members share their stories of getting off their medications and making significant progress in their health—wow! Love the website and proudly recommend *Diet Diagnosis* and the Healthnut Life Challenge—even to those I consider to be in great health. *Diet Diagnosis* and the Healthnut Life Challenge have all the ingredients in one place for you to experience your best health now! Thank you Dr. Healthnut!"

—*Pam*
Las Vegas, NV

"So excited! It's taken years for me to be intentional about making changes, at least in part because there are so many confusing and impractical systems out there. This is not a system, but a way of life that benefits the way our bodies realistically function! I've taken it seriously, have taken the intentional steps Dr. Nico recommended, and have seen great progress in just three weeks! My shopping list looks completely different. I even had headaches for days coming off of junk food, just to illustrate the effect this was having on my body. I now start with a healthy breakfast—after not having eaten breakfast for most of my adult life—and it's making a huge impact and key to a greater quality of life! I've seen such a difference in our energy levels. I love the community aspect of doing this together. *Diet Diagnosis* is awesome!

—*Claudia*
Vancouver, BC, Canada

ENDNOTES

1. Marketdata Enterprises, "Weight Loss Market in U.S. Up 1.7% to $61 Billion," PRWeb, 2013, accessed July 8, 2015, http://www.prweb.com/releases/2013/4/prweb10629316.htm.
2. L. Fontana and F. B. Hu, "Optimal body weight for health and longevity: bridging basic, clinical, and population research," *Aging Cell* 13, no. 3 (2014): 391–400, http://www.ncbi.nlm.nih.gov/pmc/articles/PMC4032609/pdf/acel0013-0391.pdf.
3. WHO, "Global status report on noncommunicable diseases," Geneva (2011):1, http://whqlibdoc.who.int/publications/2011/9789240686458_eng.pdf.

CHAPTER 1
4. "Overweight and Obesity Statistics," US Department of Health and Human Services: National Institute of Diabetes and Digestive and Kidney Diseases Web Site, accessed July 8, 2015, http://win.niddk.nih.gov/publications/PDFs/stat904z.pdf.
5. "Infographic: Public health takes on obesity," American Public Health Association, accessed July 14, 2015, http://action.apha.org/site/PageServer?pagename=Obesity_Infographic.
6. W. Zhong, et al., "Age and sex patterns of drug prescribing in a defined american population," *Mayo Clinical Procedures*, 88, no. 7 (2013): 697–707.
7. W. Wilson, MD, written communication with the author, August 1, 2013.
8. K. M. Flegal, et al., "Association of all-cause mortality with overweight and obesity using standard body mass index categories: a systematic review and meta-analysis," *JAMA*, 309, no. 1 (2013): 71–82.
9. "Obesity and Overweight," Centers for Disease Control and Prevention Web Site, accessed May 30, 2013, http://www.cdc.gov/nchs/fastats/overwt.htm.
10. "What is Epigenetics?" The University of Utah: Genetic Science Learning Center, accessed July 15, 2013, http://learn.genetics.utah.edu/content/epigenetics/.

11. D. H. Lee, et al., "Low dose organochlorine pesticides and polychlorinated biphenyls predict obesity, dyslipidemia, and insulin resistance among people free of diabetes," *PLOS ONE* 6, no. 1 (2011): e15977.

12. J. Tietelbaum, MD, oral communication with author, February 22, 2013.

13. Medline Plus, "Bone Mineral Density Scan," accessed June 18, 2013, http://www.nlm.nih.gov/medlineplus/ency/article/007197.htm.

14. J. Liang, B. E. Matheson, and K. N. Boutelle, "Neurocognitive correlates of obesity and obesity-related behaviors in children and adolescents," *International Journal of Obesity* 38, no. 4 (2014): 494–506.

15. C. Feinberg, "The Placebo Phenomenon: An ingenious researcher finds the real ingredients of 'fake' medicine," *Harvard Magazine* 1 (2013): 36–39, accessed July 15, 2013, http://harvardmag.com/pdf/2013/01-pdfs/0113-36.pdf.

16. F. J. Cronje, MD, oral communication with the author, February 22, 2013.

17. C. B. Nemeroff, "Psychoneuroimmunoendocrinology: the biological basis of mind-body physiology and pathophysiology," *Depress Anxiety* 30, no. 4 (2013): 285–287.

18. Aaron K. Vallance, "Something out of nothing: the placebo effect," *Advances in Psychiatric Treatment* 12, no. 4 (2006): 287–296; http://apt.rcpsych.org/content/aptrcpsych/12/4/287.full.pdf.

19. Harold G. Koenig, "Religion, Spirituality, and Health: The Research and Clinical Implications," *ISRN Psychiatry* (2012), http://www.ncbi.nlm.nih.gov/pmc/articles/PMC3671693/pdf/ISRN.PSYCHIATRY2012-278730.pdf.

20. D. G. Amen, *Change Your Brain, Change Your Body* (Random House Digital, 2010).

21. S. Rimer, "Happiness & Health: The biology of emotion—and what it may teach us about helping people to live longer," *Harvard School of Public Health News*, accessed July 15, 2013, http://issuu.com/harvardpublichealth/docs/hph_winter2011/.

22. Daniel Goleman, *Emotional Intelligence* (New York: Bantam Books, 1997).

23. B. Klatt, H. Murray, and M. Hiebert, *The Encyclopedia of Leadership: A practical guide to classic and contemporary leadership theories and techniques* (New York: McGraw-Hill, 2000), 455.

24. Ben Carson, *Gifted Hands: The Ben Carson Story* (Grand Rapids, MI: Zondervan, 1996).

25. "Weight Loss Market in U.S. Up 1.7% to $61 Billion," PR Web, April 16, 2013, accessed June 1, 2015, http://www.prweb.com/releases/2013/4/prweb10629316.htm.

26. L. T. Parker, MD, oral communication with the author, June 12, 2010.

CHAPTER 2

27. E. Stice, K. Burger, and S. Yokum, "Caloric deprivation increases responsivity of attention and reward brain regions to intake, anticipated intake, and images of palatable foods," *Neuroimage* 67, (2013): 322–330.

28. Coulter Jones, John Fauber, and Kristina Fiore, "Slippery slope: $$ in, diet drugs out, how five drugs came to market," *MedPage Today*, April 19, 2015, accessed July 15, 2015, http://www.medpagetoday.com/special-reports/slipperyslope/51058.

29. P. Sumithran, et al., "Long-term persistence of hormonal adaptations to weight loss," *New England Journal of Medicine* 365, no. 17 (2011): 1597–1604.

CHAPTER 3

30. B. Lundahl, et al., "Motivational interviewing in medical care settings: A systematic review and meta-analysis of randomized controlled trials," *Patient Education and Counseling* 93, no.2 (2013): 157–168.

31. Adapted from J. O. Prochaska and W. F. Velicer, "The Transtheoretical Model of Health Behavior Change," *American Journal of Health Promotion* 12, no. 1 (1997): 43, http://www.uri.edu/research/cprc/Publications/PDFs/ByTitle/The%20Transtheoretical%20model%20of%20Health%20behavior%20change.pdf.

CHAPTER 4

32. K. B. Pandey and S. I. Rizvi, "Plant polyphenols as dietary antioxidants in human health and disease," *Oxidative Medicine and Cellular Longevity* 2, no. 5 (2009): 270–278.

33. R. R. Wing and S. Phelan, "Long-term weight loss maintenance," *American Journal of Clinical Nutrition* 82, supplement 1 (2005): 222S–225S.

34. Q. Qi, et al., "Fried food consumption, genetic risk, and body mass index: gene-diet interaction analysis in three US cohort studies," *British Medical Journal* 348 (2014), http://www.ncbi.nlm.nih.gov/pmc/articles/PMC3959253/pdf/bmj.g1610.pdf.

35. J. Boone-heinonen, et al., "Fast food restaurants and food stores: longitudinal associations with diet in young to middle-aged adults: the CARDIA study," *Archives of Internal Medicine* 171, no. 13 (2011): 1162–1170.

36. I. Muraki, et al., "Rice consumption and risk of cardiovascular disease: results from a pooled analysis of 3 U.S. cohorts," *The American Journal of Clinical Nutrition* 101, no. 1 (2015): 168–170, http://www.ncbi.nlm.nih.gov/pmc/articles/PMC4266886/pdf/ajcn1011164.pdf.

37. John and Mary McDougall, *The Starch Solution* (Emmaus, PA: Rodale Books, 2013).

38. Isao Murako, et al., "Fruit consumption and risk of type 2 diabetes: results from three prospective longitudinal cohort studies," *British Medical Journal* 347 (August 29, 2013) http://www.bmj.com/content/347/bmj.f5001.

39. S. N. Bhupathiraju, et al., "Quantity and variety in fruit and vegetable intake and risk of coronary heart disease," *The American Journal of Clinical Nutrition* 98, no. 6 (2013): 151–153, http://ajcn.nutrition.org/content/98/6/1514.full.pdf+html.

40. Frank B. Hu and Walter C. Willett, "Optimal diets for prevention of coronary heart disease," *JAMA* 288, no. 20 (2002): 2575, http://isites.harvard.edu/fs/docs/icb.topic982606.files/Hu_Willett-_JAMA-_Optimal_Diets_Prevention_CHD.pdf.

41. Andreas Stengel, et al., "High-protein diet selectively reduces fat mass and improves glucose tolerance in Western-type diet-induced obese rats," *American Journal of Physiology* 305, no. 6 (2013): 582–591, http://www.ncbi.nlm.nih.gov/pmc/articles/PMC3763043/?report=reader.

42. Robert Atkins, *Dr. Atkins' New Diet Revolution* (New York: Harper; 2009).

43. A. Astrup, A. Raben, and N. Geiker, "The role of higher protein diets in weight control and obesity-related comorbidities," *International Journal of Obesity* 39, no. 5 (2015): 722, http://www.ncbi.nlm.nih.gov/pmc/articles/PMC4424378/pdf/ijo2014216a.pdf.

44. A. M. Bernstein, et al., "Major Dietary Protein Sources and the Risk of Coronary Heart Disease in Women," *Circulation* 122, no. 9 (2010): 876–883, http://www.ncbi.nlm.nih.gov/pmc/articles/PMC2946797/pdf/nihms-229256.pdf.

45. L. De Koning, et al., "Low-carbohydrate diet scores and risk of type 2 diabetes in men," *The American Journal of Clinical Nutrition* 93, no. 4 (2011): 844–850,http://www.ncbi.nlm.nih.gov/pmc/articles/PMC3057550/pdf/ajcn9340844.pdf.

46. M. Harvie, et al., "The effect of intermittent energy and carbohydrate restriction v. daily energy restriction on weight loss and metabolic disease risk markers in overweight women," *British Journal of Nutrition* 110 (2013): 1534–1547.

47. H. M. Dashti, et al., "Long-term effects of a ketogenic diet in obese patients," *Experimental & Clinical Cardiology* 9, no. 3 (2004): 203, http://www.ncbi.nlm.nih.gov/pmc/articles/PMC2716748/pdf/ecc09200.pdf.

48. A. Paoli, "Ketogenic Diet for Obesity: Friend or Foe?" *International Journal of Environmental Research and Public Health* 11, no. 2 (2014): 2097, http://www.ncbi.nlm.nih.gov/pmc/articles/PMC3945587/pdf/ijerph-11-02092.pdf.

49. Mary Enig and Sally Fallon, *Eat Fat, Lose Fat* (New York: Plume, 2006).

50. Frank B. Hu, et al., "Frequent nut consumption and risk of coronary heart disease in women: prospective cohort study," *British Medical Journal* 217 (1998): 1341–1345, http://www.ncbi.nlm.nih.gov/pmc/articles/PMC28714/pdf/1341.pdf.

51. Y. Bao, et al., "Association of Nut Consumption with Total and Cause-Specific Mortality," *The New England Journal of Medicine* 369, no. 21 (2013): 2001–2011, http://www.ncbi.nlm.nih.gov/pmc/articles/PMC3931001/pdf/nihms552688.pdf.

52. V. Garneau, I. Rudkowska, and A. M. Paradis, "Association between plasma omega-3 fatty acids and cardiovascular disease risk factors," *Applied Physiology, Nutrition, and Metabolism* 38, no. 3 (2013): 243–248.

53. "Fats and Cholesterol: Out with the Bad, In with the Good," Harvard School of Public Health: The Nutrition Source Website, accessed July 25, 2013, http://www.hsph.harvard.edu/nutritionsource/fats-full-story/.

54. M. Fogelholm, et al., "Dietary macronutrients and food consumption as determinants of long-term weight change in adult populations: a systematic literature review," *Food & Nutrition* Research 56, (2012): 10, http://www.ncbi.nlm.nih.gov/pmc/articles/PMC3418611/pdf/FNR-56-19103.pdf.

CHAPTER 5

55. T. Colin Campbell and Thomas M. Campbell, *The China Study* (Dallas, Texas: BenBella Books, 2006).

56. S. Agrawal, et al., "Type of vegetarian diet, obesity and diabetes in adult Indian population," *Nutrition Journal* 13 (2014): 89, http://www.ncbi.nlm.nih.gov/pmc/articles/PMC4168165/.

57. T. M. Campbell and T. C. Campbell, "The benefits of integrating nutrition into clinical medicine," *The Israel Medical Association Journal* 10, no. 10 (2008): 730–732.

58. Y. Yokoyama, et al., "Vegetarian diets and glycemic control in diabetes: a systematic review and meta-analysis," *Cardiovascular Diagnosis and Therapy* 4, no. 5 (2014): 373–382, http://www.ncbi.nlm.nih.gov/pmc/articles/PMC4221319/pdf/cdt-04-05-373.pdf.

59. For more information, visit http://www.huffingtonpost.com/craig-cooper/soy-and-chocolate-too-muc_b_756604.html.

60. Frank Newport, "In U.S., 5% Consider Themselves Vegetarian," Gallup: Well-being, July 26, 2012, http://www.gallup.com/poll/156215/consider-themselves-vegetarians.aspx.

61. L. T. Le and J. Sabaté, "Beyond Meatless, the Health Effects of Vegan Diets: Findings from the Adventist Cohorts," *Nutrients* 6, no. 6 (2014): 2131–2147, http://www.ncbi.nlm.nih.gov/pmc/articles/PMC4073139/pdf/nutrients-06-02131.pdf.

62. Joel Fuhrman, *Eat to Live* (Boston: Little, Brown and Company, 2011).

63. M. Glick-Bauer and M-C Yeh, "The Health Advantage of a Vegan Diet: Exploring the Gut Microbiota Connection," *Nutrients* 6, no. 11 (2014): 4832–4833, http://www.ncbi.nlm.nih.gov/pmc/articles/PMC4245565/pdf/nutrients-06-04822.pdf.

64. For more information on the Blue Zone, visit http://www.npr.org/sections/thesalt/2015/04/11/398325030/eating-to-break-100-longevity-diet-tips-from-the-blue-zones.

65. K. S. Woo, et al., "Vegan Diet, Subnormal Vitamin B-12 Status and Cardiovascular Health," *Nutrients* 6, no. 8 (2014): 3259–3273, http://www.ncbi.nlm.nih.gov/pmc/articles/PMC4145307/pdf/nutrients-06-03259.pdf.

66. P. J. Tuso, et al., "Nutritional Update for Physicians: Plant-Based Diets," *The Permanente Journal* 17, no. 2 (2013): 62.

67. J. R. Knurick, "Comparison of Correlates of Bone Mineral Density in Individuals Adhering to Lacto-Ovo, Vegan, or Omnivore Diets: A Cross-Sectional Investigation," *Nutrients* 7, no. 5 (2015): 3416–3426, http://www.ncbi.nlm.nih.gov/pmc/articles/PMC4446759/pdf/nutrients-07-03416.pdf.

68. F. Fallucca, "Gut microbiota and Ma-Pi 2 macrobiotic diet in the treatment of type 2 diabetes," *World Journal of Diabetes* 6, no. 3 (2015): 403–411, http://www.ncbi.nlm.nih.gov/pmc/articles/PMC4398897/pdf/WJD-6-403.pdf.

69. A. Soare, et al., "The effect of the macrobiotic Ma-Pi 2 diet vs. the recommended diet in the management of type 2 diabetes: the randomized controlled MADIAB trial," *Nutrition & Metabolism* 11 (2014): 39, http://www.ncbi.nlm.nih.gov/pmc/articles/PMC4190933/pdf/1743-7075-11-39.pdf.

70. J. M. Lattimer and M. D. Haub, "Effects of Dietary Fiber and Its Components on Metabolic Health," *Nutrients* 2, no. 12 (2010): 1281, http://www.ncbi.nlm.nih.gov/pmc/articles/PMC3257631/pdf/nutrients-02-01266.pdf.

71. J. Slavin, "Fiber and Prebiotics: Mechanisms and Health Benefits," *Nutrients* 5, no. 4 (2013): 1417–1435, http://www.ncbi.nlm.nih.gov/pmc/articles/PMC3705355/pdf/nutrients-05-01417.pdf.

72. K. N. Grooms, "Dietary Fiber Intake and Cardiometabolic Risks among US Adults, NHANES 1999–2010," *The American Journal of Medicine* 126, no. 12 (2013): http://www.ncbi.nlm.nih.gov/pmc/articles/PMC3865784/pdf/nihms531655.pdf.

73. A. J. Lanou and B. Svenson, "Reduced cancer risk in vegetarians: an analysis of recent reports," *Cancer Management and Research* 3 (2011): 7, http://www.ncbi.nlm.nih.gov/pmc/articles/PMC3048091/pdf/cmr-3-001.pdf.

74. Q. Chan, et al., "Relation of raw and cooked vegetable consumption to blood pressure: the INTERMAP Study," *Journal of Human Hypertension* 28, no. 6 (2014): 353, http://www.ncbi.nlm.nih.gov/pmc/articles/PMC4013197/pdf/jhh2013115a.pdf.

75. V. D. Longo and M. P. Mattson, "Fasting: Molecular Mechanisms and Clinical Applications," *Cell Metabolism* 19, no. 2 (2014): 181–192, http://www.ncbi.nlm.nih.gov/pmc/articles/PMC3946160/pdf/nihms551820.pdf.

76. D. N. Lavin, et al., "Fasting induces an anti-inflammatory effect on the neuroimmune system which a high-fat diet prevents," *Obesity* 19, no. 8 (2011): 1587, http://www.ncbi.nlm.nih.gov/pmc/articles/PMC3695639/pdf/nihms-480815.pdf.

77. For the biblical account of the prophet Daniel, see Daniel 1:8–14; 10:2–3.

78. J. F. Trepanowski and R. J. Bloomer, "The impact of religious fasting on human health," *Nutrition Journal* 9 (2010): 57, http://www.ncbi.nlm.nih.gov/pmc/articles/PMC2995774/pdf/1475-2891-9-57.pdf.

79. K. A. Varady, et al., "Alternate day fasting for weight loss in normal weight and overweight subjects: a randomized controlled trial," *Nutrition Journal* 12 (2013): 146, http://www.ncbi.nlm.nih.gov/pmc/articles/PMC3833266/pdf/1475-2891-12-146.pdf.

80. Michael Mosley and Mimi Spencer, *The Fast Diet* (New York: Atria, 2013).

81. K. K. Hoddy, et al., "Safety of alternate day fasting and effect on disordered eating behaviors," *Nutrition Journal* 14 (2015): 44, http://www.ncbi.nlm.nih.gov/pmc/articles/PMC4424827/pdf/12937_2015_Article_29.pdf.

82. O. T. Mytton, "Systematic review and meta-analysis of the effect of increased vegetable and fruit consumption on body weight and energy intake," *BMC Public Health* 14 (2014): 886, http://www.ncbi.nlm.nih.gov/pmc/articles/PMC4158137/pdf/12889_2014_Article_7014.pdf.

83. S. F. Shenoy, et al., "Weight loss in individuals with metabolic syndrome given DASH diet counseling when provided a low sodium vegetable juice: a randomized controlled trial," *Nutrition Journal* 9 (2010): 8, http://www.ncbi.nlm.nih.gov/pmc/articles/PMC2841082/pdf/1475-2891-9-8.pdf.

84. Alejandro Junger, MD, *Clean* (New York: HarperOne, 2012).

85. J. L. Barger, R. L. Walford, and R. Weindruch, "The retardation of aging by caloric restriction: its significance in the transgenic era," *Experimental Gerontology* 38, no. 11–12 (2003): 1343–1351.

86. J. F. Trepanowski, et al., "Impact of caloric and dietary restriction regimens on markers of health and longevity in humans and animals: a summary of available findings," *Nutrition Journal* 10 (2011): 107, http://www.ncbi.nlm.nih.gov/pmc/articles/PMC3200169/pdf/1475-2891-10-107.pdf.

87. L. Fontana and F. B. Hu, "Optimal body weight for health and longevity: bridging basic, clinical, and population research," *Aging Cell* 13, no. 3 (2014): 395, http://www.ncbi.nlm.nih.gov/pmc/articles/PMC4032609/pdf/acel0013-0391.pdf.

88. E. Cava and L. Fontana, "Will calorie restriction work in humans?" *Aging* 5, no. 7 (2013): 507, http://www.ncbi.nlm.nih.gov/pmc/articles/PMC3765579/pdf/aging-05-507.pdf.

89. E. Lopez-Garcia, et al., "The Mediterranean-style dietary pattern and mortality among men and women with cardiovascular disease," *The American Journal of Clinical Nutrition* 99, no. 1 (2014): 172, http://www.ncbi.nlm.nih.gov/pmc/articles/PMC3862454/pdf/ajcn991172.pdf.

90. F. Sofi, "Adherence to Mediterranean diet and health status: meta-analysis," *British Medical Journal* 333 (2008), http://www.ncbi.nlm.nih.gov/pmc/articles/PMC2533524/pdf/bmj.a1344.pdf.

91. E. Lopez-Garcia, et al., "The Mediterranean-style dietary pattern and mortality among men and women with cardiovascular disease," *The American Journal of Clinical Nutrition* 99, no. 1 (2014): 178, http://www.ncbi.nlm.nih.gov/pmc/articles/PMC3862454/pdf/ajcn991172.pdf.

92. D. Mozaffarian, et al., "Plasma phospholipid long-chain fatty acids and total and cause-specific mortality in older adults: a cohort study," *Annals of Internal Medicine* 158, no. 7 (2013): 515–525.

93. Annia Ciezadlo "Does the Mediterranean Diet Even Exist?" *The New York Times*, April 1, 2011, accessed June 26, 2015, http://www.nytimes.com/2011/04/03/magazine/mag-03YouRHere-t.html?_r=2&.

94. E. García-Fernández, et al., "A. Mediterranean Diet and Cardiodiabesity: A Review," *Nutrients* 6, no. 9 (2014): 3474, http://www.ncbi.nlm.nih.gov/pmc/articles/PMC4179172/pdf/nutrients-06-03474.pdf.

95. D, C, Klonoff, "The Beneficial Effects of a Paleolithic Diet on Type 2 Diabetes and Other Risk Factors for Cardiovascular Disease," *Journal of Diabetes Science and Technology* 3, no. 6 (2009): 1229–1232, http://www.ncbi.nlm.nih.gov/pmc/articles/PMC2787021/pdf/dst-03-1229.pdf.

96. T. Jönsson, et al., "A paleolithic diet is more satiating per calorie than a mediterranean-like diet in individuals with ischemic heart disease," *Nutrition & Metabolism* 7 (2010): 85, http://www.ncbi.nlm.nih.gov/pmc/articles/PMC3009971/pdf/1743-7075-7-85.pdf.

97. C. Mellberg, et al., "Long-term effects of a Palaeolithic-type diet in obese postmenopausal women: a two-year randomized trial," *European Journal of Clinical Nutrition* 68, no. 3 (2014): 350–357, http://www.ncbi.nlm.nih.gov/pmc/articles/PMC4216932/pdf/emss-60632.pdf.

98. I. Spreadbury, "Comparison with ancestral diets suggests dense acellular carbohydrates promote an inflammatory microbiota, and may be the primary dietary cause of leptin resistance and obesity," *Journal of Diabetes, Metabolic Syndrome and Obesity* 5 (2012): 175–189.

99. G. Frost, et al., "The short-chain fatty acid acetate reduces appetite via a central homeostatic mechanism," *Nature Communications*, April 29, 2014 (online), supplementary information available for this article at http://www.nature.com/ncomms/2014/140429/ncomms4611/suppinfo/ncomms4611_S1.html.

100. T. Jönsson, et al., "Beneficial effects of a Paleolithic diet on cardiovascular risk factors in type 2 diabetes: a randomized cross-over pilot study," *Cardiovascular Diabetology* 8 (2009): 35, http://www.ncbi.nlm.nih.gov/pmc/articles/PMC2724493/pdf/1475-2840-8-35.pdf.

CHAPTER 6

101. Tana Amen, *The Omni Diet* (New York: St. Martin's Press, 2013).

102. G. S. Frost, et al., "Impacts of Plant-Based Foods in Ancestral Hominin Diets on the Metabolism and Function of Gut Microbiota In Vitro," *MBio* 5, no. 3 (2014), http://www.ncbi.nlm.nih.gov/pmc/articles/PMC4030449/pdf/mBio.00853-14.pdf.

103. S. L. Schnorr, et al., "Gut microbiome of the Hadza hunter-gatherers," *Nature Communications* 5 (2014): 3654, http://www.ncbi.nlm.nih.gov/pmc/articles/PMC3996546/pdf/ncomms4654.pdf.

104. George Malkmus and Peter Shockey, *The Hallelujah Diet* (Shippensburg, PA: Destiny, 2006).

105. M. S. Donaldson, N. Speight, S. Loomis, "Fibromyalgia syndrome improved using a mostly raw vegetarian diet: An observational study," *BMC Complementary and Alternative Medicine* 1, (2001): 7, http://www.ncbi.nlm.nih.gov/pmc/articles/PMC57816/pdf/1472-6882-1-7.pdf.

106. M. S. Donaldson, "Nutrition and cancer: A review of the evidence for an anti-cancer diet," *Nutrition Journal* 3 (2004), http://www.ncbi.nlm.nih.gov/pmc/articles/PMC526387/.

107. Jordan S. Rubin, *The Maker's Diet* (Shippensburg, PA: Destiny, 2013).

108. H. H. Murphy, "Biblical Medicine and Hygiene," *Canadian Medical Association Journal* 22, no. 2 (1930): 263, http://www.ncbi.nlm.nih.gov/pmc/articles/ PMC381729/pdf/canmedaj00089-0106.pdf.

109. See 1 Timothy 4:4.

110. See 1 Corinthians 10:23.

111. S. L. Vieille, et al., "Estimated Levels of Gluten Incidentally Present in a Canadian Gluten-Free Diet," *Nutrients* 6, no. 2 (2014): 882, http://www.ncbi. nlm.nih.gov/pmc/articles/PMC3942737/pdf/nutrients-06-00881.pdf.

112. William Davis, MD, *Wheat Belly* (Emmaus, PA: Rodale, 2014).

113. L. Saturni, G. Ferretti, and T. Bacchetti, "The Gluten-Free Diet: Safety and Nutritional Quality," *Nutrients* 2, no. 1 (2010): 20–21, http://www.ncbi.nlm. nih.gov/pmc/articles/PMC3257612/pdf/nutrients-02-00016.pdf.

114. G. Mazzarella, et al., "Reintroduction of gluten following flour transamidation in adult celiac patients: a randomized, controlled clinical study," *Journal of Clinical and Development Immunology* (online) 2012, http://dx.doi. org/10.1155/2012/329150.

115. Y. Sanz, "Effects of a gluten-free diet on gut microbiota and immune function in healthy adult humans," *Landes Bioscience* 1, no. 3 (2010): 135–137.

116. A. Diamanti, et al., "Celiac Disease and Overweight in Children: An Update," *Nutrients* 6, no. 1 (2014): 211–214, http://www.ncbi.nlm.nih.gov/pmc/articles/ PMC3916856/pdf/nutrients-06-00207.pdf.

117. J. L. Buell, et al., "Presence of Metabolic Syndrome in Football Linemen," *Journal of Athletic Training* 43, no. 6 (2008): 608–615, http://www.ncbi.nlm. nih.gov/pmc/articles/PMC2582553/pdf/attr-43-06-608.pdf.

118. R. Leischik and N. Spelsberg, "Vegan Triple-Ironman (Raw Vegetables/ Fruits)," *Case Reports in Cardiology* (2014), http://www.ncbi.nlm.nih.gov/pmc/ articles/PMC4008446/pdf/CRIM.CARDIOLOGY2014-317246.pdf.

119. C. B. Becker, et al., "Can we reduce eating disorder risk factors in female college athletes?" *Body Image* 9, no. 1 (2012): 31–42.

120. E. R. Christ, et al., "The effect of increased lipid intake on hormonal responses during aerobic exercise in endurance-trained men," *European Journal of Endocrinology* 154, no. 3 (2006): 397–403.

121. Bill Phillips, *Body for Life* (New York: Harper Collins, 1998).

122. S. L. Halson, "Sleep in Elite Athletes and Nutritional Interventions to Enhance Sleep," *Sports Medicine* (Auckland, NZ) 44 (2014): 13–23, http://www.ncbi. nlm.nih.gov/pmc/articles/PMC4008810/pdf/40279_2014_Article_147.pdf.

123. F. M. Sacks, et al., "Comparison of weight-loss diets with different compositions of fat, protein, and carbohydrates," *New England Journal of Medicine* 360, no. 9 (2009): 859–873.

124. D.L. Katz1 and S. Meller, "Can We Say What Diet Is Best for Health?" *Annual Review of Public Health* 35 (2014): 83–103, http://www.annualreviews. org/doi/full/10.1146/annurev-publhealth-032013-182351.

125. J. B. German, et al., "Nutrigenomics and Personalized Diets: What Will They Mean for Food?" *Annual Review of Food, Science, and Technology* 2 (2011): 97–123, http://www.ncbi.nlm.nih.gov/pmc/articles/PMC4414021/pdf/nihms671182.pdf.

126. For more information on Dr. Roizen's strategy, visit his ebook at http://www.amazon.com/This-Is-Your-Do-Over-Secrets-ebook/dp/B00P42WPVQ, 128-130.

127. See https://www.bostonglobe.com/opinion/2015/03/11/that-new-report-cholesterol-actually-kind-old-news/xAV02K8lT46t77U4FY7e2I/story.html.

CHAPTER 7

128. K. De Punder and L. Pruimboom, "Stress Induces Endotoxemia and Low-Grade Inflammation by Increasing Barrier Permeability," *Frontiers in Immunology* 6 (2015): 223, http://www.ncbi.nlm.nih.gov/pmc/articles/PMC4432792/pdf/fimmu-06-00223.pdf.

129. G. Egger and J. Dixon, "Beyond Obesity and Lifestyle: A Review of 21st Century Chronic Disease Determinants," *BioMed Research International* (2014), http://www.ncbi.nlm.nih.gov/pmc/articles/PMC3997940/pdf/BMRI2014-731685.pdf.

130. "Obesity and Overweight," Centers for Disease Control and Prevention Web Site, accessed May 30, 2013, http://www.cdc.gov/nchs/fastats/overwt.htm.

131. Garry Gordon, MD, email communication with the author, May 15, 2012.

132. M. G. Weisskopf, et al., "A prospective study of bone lead concentration and death from all causes, cardiovascular diseases, and cancer," *Department of Veterans Affairs Normative Aging Study* 120, no. 12 (2009): 1056–1064.

133. O. Lee, et al., "Fructose and carbonyl metabolites as endogenous toxins," *Chemico-Biological Interactions* 178, no. 1–3 (2009): 332–339.

134. "Body Burden: The Pollution in Newborns," Environmental Working Group Web site, accessed July 16, 2013, http://www.ewg.org/research/body-burden-pollution-newborns.

CHAPTER 8

135. "Frequently Asked Questions on Genenitically Modified Foods," World Health Organization, accessed July 20, 2015, http://www.who.int/foodsafety/areas_work/food-technology/faq-genetically-modified-food/en/.

136. For more information on why the consumption of GM food is so widespread, see this informative study from Friends of the Earth International: http://www.foeeurope.org/sites/default/files/publications/foei_who_benefits_from_gm_crops_2014.pdf.

137. M. Antoniou, C. Robinson, and J. Fagan, "GMO Myths and Truths: An evidence-based examination of the claims made for the safety and efficacy of genetically modified crops," Earth Open Source Web site, accessed July 20, 2015, http://gmomythsandtruths.earthopensource.org/.

138. For more information, visit http://www.nongmoproject.org/learn-more/what-is-gmo/.

139. Ibid.

140. A. S. Bawa and K. R. Anilakumar, "Genetically modified foods: safety, risks and public concerns—a review," *Journal of Food, Science, and Technology* 50, no. 6 (2013): 1035–1036.

141. M. Cuhra, T. Traavik, and T. Bohn, "Clone- and age-dependent toxicity of a glyphosate commercial formulation and its active ingredient in Daphnia magna," *Ecotoxicology* 22, no. 2 (2013): 251–262.

142. Kathryn C. Guyton, et al., "Carcinogenicity of tetrachlorvinphos, parathion, malathion, diazinon, and glyphosate," *The Lancet Oncology* 16, no. 5 (2015): 490–491, http://www.thelancet.com/pdfs/journals/lanonc/PIIS1470-2045(15)70134-8.pdf.

143. S. Thongprakaisang, et al., "Glyphosate induces human breast cancer cells growth via estrogen receptors," *Journal of Food and Chemical Toxicology* 59 (2013): 129–136.

144. G. E. Séralini, et al, "Long term toxicity of a Roundup herbicide and a Roundup-tolerant genetically modified maize," *Journal of Food and Chemical Toxicology* 50, no. 11 (2012): 4221–4231.

145. M. Antoniou, C. Robinson, and J. Fagan, "GMO Myths and Truths: An evidence-based examination of the claims made for the safety and efficacy of genetically modified crops," Earth Open Source Web site, accessed July 20, 2015, http://gmomythsandtruths.earthopensource.org/.

146. To see the report, visit http://www.gifsoja.nl/Gifsoja/nieuws/Artikelen/2012/12/15_Reclame_Code_Commissie__Roundup_advertentie_Monsanto_is_misleidend_files/Uitspraak%20RCC%20Monsanto%20Roundup%20advertentie%20121211.pdf.

147. For more information on Netherland's actions against glyphosate, visit http://sustainablepulse.com/2014/04/04/dutch-parliament-bans-glyphosate-herbicides-non-commercial-use/ (accessed July 8, 2015).

148. A. Samsel and S. Seneff, "Glyphosate's Suppression of Cytochrome P450 Enzymes and Amino Acid Biosynthesis by the Gut Microbiome: Pathways to Modern Diseases," *Entropy* 15, no. 4 (2013): 1416.

149. Ross Pelton, James B. LaValle, and Ernest B. Hawkins, *Drug-Induced Nutrient Depletion Handbook* (Hudson, Ohio: Lexi-Comp, Inc, 2001).

150. See http://www.gmaonline.org/news-events/newsroom/FactsAboutGMOs/.

151. Anna Almendrala, "Prop 37 Defeated: California Voters Reject Mandatory GMO-Labeling," *The Huffington Post*, accessed July 16, 2013, http://www.huffingtonpost.com/2012/11/07/prop-37-defeated-californ_n_2088402.html.

152. Michael McAuliff, "GMO Labeling Bill Voted Down In Senate," *The Huffington Post*, accessed February 15, 2014, http://www.huffingtonpost.com/2013/05/23/gmo-labeling-bill-genetically-modified-food_n_3325972.html.

153. Christopher Doering, "Mandatory GM Food Labeling," *USA TODAY*, July 14, 2015, accessed July 21, 2015, http://www.usatoday.com/story/news/nation/2015/07/14/house-committee-passes-bill-to-ban-states-from-requiring-gmo-food-labeling/30141681/.

154. Ryan Villarreal, "Not Entirely Organic: Whole Foods to Label All GMO Products by 2018," *International Business Times*, accessed 16 July 2013, http://www.ibtimes.com/not-entirely-organic-whole-foods-label-all-gmo-products-2018-1175421.

155. See http://www.centerforfoodsafety.org/issues/309/ge-fish#.

CHAPTER 9

156. B. M. Popkin, L. S. Adiar, S. W. Ng, "Now and Then: The Global Nutrition Transition: The Pandemic of Obesity in Developing Countries," *Nutrition Review* 70, no. 1 (2012): 3–21, http://www.ncbi.nlm.nih.gov/pmc/articles/PMC3257829/pdf/nihms336201.pdf.

157. J. P. Karl and E. Saltzman, "The role of whole grains in body weight regulation," *Advanced Nutrition* 3, no. 5 (2012): 697–707.

158. S. C. Lucan, A. Karpyn, and S. Sherman, "Storing Empty Calories and Chronic Disease Risk: Snack-Food Products, Nutritive Content, and Manufacturers in Philadelphia Corner Stores," *Journal of Urban Health : Bulletin of the New York Academy of Medicine* 87, no. 3 (2010): 400–402, http://www.ncbi.nlm.nih.gov/pmc/articles/PMC2871092/pdf/11524_2010_Article_9453.pdf.

159. D. Yu, et al., "Dietary Carbohydrates, Refined Grains, Glycemic Load, and Risk of Coronary Heart Disease in Chinese Adults," *American Journal of Epidemiology* 178, no. 10 (2013): 1544–1545, http://www.ncbi.nlm.nih.gov/pmc/articles/PMC3888273/pdf/kwt178.pdf.

160. For an example of this being documented on a specific people group, see M. Kristensen, et al., "Whole grain compared with refined wheat decreases the percentage of body fat following a 12-week, energy-restricted dietary intervention in postmenopausal women," *Journal of Nutrition* 142, no. 4 (2012): 710–716.

161. X. Shang, et al., "Dietary pattern and its association with the prevalence of obesity and related cardiometabolic risk factors among Chinese children," *PLOS ONE* 7, no. 8 (2012): e43183.

162. V. Mohan, et al., "Effect of Brown Rice, White Rice, and Brown Rice with Legumes on Blood Glucose and Insulin Responses in Overweight Asian Indians: A Randomized Controlled Trial," *Diabetes Technology & Therapeutics* 16, no. 5 (2014): 321, http://www.ncbi.nlm.nih.gov/pmc/articles/PMC3996977/pdf/dia.2013.0259.pdf.

163. Q. Sun, et al., "White Rice, Brown Rice, and Risk of Type 2 Diabetes in US Men and Women," *Archives of Internal Medicine* 170, no. 11 (2010): 965, http://www.ncbi.nlm.nih.gov/pmc/articles/PMC3024208/pdf/nihms261139.pdf.

164. Z. Li, et al., "Pistachio nuts reduce triglycerides and body weight by comparison to refined carbohydrate snack in obese subjects on a 12-week weight loss program," *Journal of the American College of Nutrition* 29, no. 3 (2010): 198–203.

165. J. T. Dwyer, et al., "Is 'Processed' a Four-Letter Word? The Role of Processed Foods in Achieving Dietary Guidelines and Nutrient Recommendations," *Advances in Nutrition* 3 (2012): 538, http://www.ncbi.nlm.nih.gov/pmc/articles/PMC3649724/pdf/536.pdf.

166. Mark Hyman, *The Blood Sugar Solution* (New York: Little, Brown and Company, 2012).

167. Robert Lustig, *Fat Chance* (New York: Hudson Street Press, 2012).

168. S. Boseley, "Sugar, not fat, exposed as deadly villain in obesity epidemic," *The Guardian*, March 20, 2013, accessed July 16, 2013, http://www.guardian.co.uk/society/2013/mar/20/sugar-deadly-obesity-epidemic.

169. J. C. Moubarac, et al., "Consumption of ultra-processed foods and likely impact on human health," Public Health Nutrition 16, no. 12 (2013): 2240–2248.

170. L. I. Lesser, F. J. Zimmerman, and D. A. Cohen, "Outdoor advertising, obesity, and soda consumption: a cross-sectional study," *BMC Public Health* 13, no. 1 (2013): 20.

171. C. Relton, M. Strong, M. Holdsworth, "Plastic food packaging encourages obesity," *BMJ* 344, no. 1 (2012): e3824.

172. Michael Moss, "The Extraordinary Science of Addictive Junk Food," *The New York Times*, February 20, 2013, accessed July 16, 2013, http://www.nytimes.com/2013/02/24/magazine/the-extraordinary-science-of-junk-food.html?pagewanted=all&_r=2&.

173. L. Claudio, "Our food: packaging & public health," *Environmental Health Perspective* 120, no. 6 (2012): A232–237.

174. I. Borgmeier and J. Westenhoefer, "Impact of different food label formats on healthiness evaluation and food choice of consumers: a randomized-controlled study," *BMC Public Health* 9 (2009), http://www.ncbi.nlm.nih.gov/pmc/articles/PMC2702386/.

CHAPTER 10

175. L. Oates and M. Cohen, "Assessing Diet as a Modifiable Risk Factor for Pesticide Exposure," *International Journal of Environmental Research and Public Health* 8, no. 6 (2011): 1793, http://www.ncbi.nlm.nih.gov/pmc/articles/PMC3137997/pdf/ijerph-08-01792.pdf.

176. E. Johansson, et al., "Contribution of Organically Grown Crops to Human Health," *International Journal of Environmental Research and Public Health* 11, no. 4 (2014): 3870–3893, http://www.ncbi.nlm.nih.gov/pmc/articles/PMC4025038/pdf/ijerph-11-03870.pdf.

177. S. Watson "Organic food no more nutritious than conventionally grown food," *Harvard Health Publications*, http://www.health.harvard.edu/blog/organic-food-no-more-nutritious-than-conventionally-grown-food-201209055264.

178. K. Everstine, J. Spink, and S. Kennedy, "Economically motivated adulteration (EMA) of food: common characteristics of EMA incidents," *Journal of Food Protection* 76, no. 4 (2013): 723–735.

179. "Faux pas! Food fraud on the rise," *CNN*, January 23, 2013, accessed July 16, 2013, http://eatocracy.cnn.com/2013/01/23/faux-pas-food-fraud-on-the-rise/.

CHAPTER 11

180. S. Connor, "Overeating and obesity to blame for medical disorders, not plastics chemical found in body," *The Independent*, February 15, 2013, accessed July 16, 2013, http://www.independent.co.uk/news/science/overeating-and-obesity-to-blame-for-medical-disorders-not-plastics-chemical-found-in-body-8497131.html.

181. D. Barry, M. Clarke, and N. M. Petry, "Obesity and its relationship to addictions: is overeating a form of addictive behavior?" *American Journal on Addictions* 18, no. 6 (2009): 439–451.

182. A. Kong, et al., "Adoption of diet-related self-monitoring behaviors varies by race/ethnicity, education, and baseline binge eating score among overweight-to-obese postmenopausal women in a 12-month dietary weight loss intervention," *Nutrition Research* 32, no. 4 (2012): 260–265.

183. L. H. Epstein, et al., "Long-term habituation to food in obese and nonobese women," *American Journal of Clinical Nutrition* 94, no. 2 (2011): 371–376.

184. M. Marchione and M. Stobbe, "Fructose Linked to Overeating, Obesity in New Brain Imaging Study," *The Huffington Post*, January 2, 2013, accessed July 16, 2013, http://www.huffingtonpost.com/2013/01/02/fructose-overeating-obesity-brain-imaging-_n_2395413.html.

185. E. J. McAllister, et al., "Ten Putative Contributors to the Obesity Epidemic," *Critical Reviews in Food, Science, and Nutrition* 49, no. 10 (2009): 871, http://www.ncbi.nlm.nih.gov/pmc/articles/PMC2932668/pdf/nihms225558.pdf.

186. Z. Cooper, et al., "Testing a new cognitive behavioural treatment for obesity: A randomized controlled trial with three-year follow-up," *Behavioral Research Therapy* 48, no. 8 (2010): 706–713.

CHAPTER 12

187. R. E. Larraín, et al., "Finishing steers with diets based on corn, high-tannin sorghum, or a mix of both: feedlot performance, carcass characteristics, and beef sensory attributes," *Journal of Animal Science* 87, no. 6 (2009): 2089–2095.

188. M. A. Valvo, et al., "Effect of ewe feeding system (grass v. concentrate) on intramuscular fatty acids of lambs raised exclusively on maternal milk," *ASC* 81, no. 3 (2005).

189. C. A. Daley, et al., "A review of fatty acid profiles and antioxidant content in grass-fed and grain-fed beef," *Nutrition Journal* 9 (2010): 10.

190. P. E. Miller, et al., "Meat-related compounds and colorectal cancer risk by anatomical subsite," *Nutrition and Cancer* 65, no. 2 (2013): 202–226.

191. B. Aschebrook-kilfoy, X. O. Shu, Y. T. Gao, et al., "Thyroid cancer risk and dietary nitrate and nitrite intake in the Shanghai women's health study," *International Journal of Cancer* 132, no. 4 (2013): 897–904.

192. For more information, visit http://www.thyroidawareness.com/.

193. V. Dhaka, et al., "Trans fats-sources, health risks and alternative approach - A review," *Journal of Food, Science, and Technology* 48, no. 5 (2011): 534–541.

194. Z. Kochan, J. Karbowska, E. Babicz-zielińska, "[Dietary trans-fatty acids and metabolic syndrome]" *Postepy Hig Med Dosw* [article in Polish] 64 (2010): 650–658.

195. "Shining the Spotlight on Trans Fats," *Harvard Public Health Nutrition*, accessed July 16, 2013, http://www.hsph.harvard.edu/nutritionsource/transfats/.

196. Jonny Bowden and Stephen Sinatra, *The Great Cholesterol Myth* (Beverly, MA: Fair Winds Press, 2012).

197. M. Dhibi, et al., "The intake of high fat diet with different trans fatty acid levels differentially induces oxidative stress and non-alcoholic fatty liver disease (NAFLD) in rats," *Nutrition & Metabolism* 8, no. 1 (2011): 65.

198. S. N. Han, et al., "Effect of hydrogenated and saturated, relative to polyunsaturated, fat on immune and inflammatory responses of adults with moderate hypercholesterolemia," *Journal of Lipid Research* 43, no. 3 (2002): 445–452.

199. S. Couvreur, et al., "The Linear Relationship Between the Proportion of Fresh Grass in the Cow Diet, Milk Fatty Acid Composition, and Butter Properties," *Journal of Dairy Science* 89, no. 6 (2006): 1956–1969.

200. S. Kobylewski and M. F. Jacobson, "Toxicology of food dyes," *International Journal of Occupational and Environmental Health* 18, no. 3 (2012): 220–246.

201. L. P. Sycheva, et al., "Investigation of genotoxic and cytotoxic effects of micro- and nanosized titanium dioxide in six organs of mice in vivo," *Mutational Research* 726, no. 1 (2011): 8–14.

202. J. He and M. M. Giusti, "Anthocyanins: natural colorants with health-promoting properties," *Annual Review of Food, Science and Technology* 1, no. 1 (2010): 163–187.

203. "Names of ingredients that contain processed free glutamic acid (MSG)," Truth in Labeling, accessed July 17, 2013, http://www.truthinlabeling.org/hiddensources.html.

204. O. A. Rotimi, et al., "Effects of fibre-enriched diets on tissue lipid profiles of MSG obese rats," *Food and Chemical Toxicology* 50, no. 11 (2012): 4062–4067.

205. K. S. Collison, et al., "Dietary trans-fat combined with monosodium glutamate induces dyslipidemia and impairs spatial memory," *Physiology & Behavior* 99, no. 3 (2010): 334–342.

206. For more information, visit: http://www.truthinlabeling.org/nomsg.html (accessed July 17, 2013).

CHAPTER 13

207. M. I. Goran, S. J. Ulijaszek, and E. E. Ventura, "High fructose corn syrup and diabetes prevalence: a global perspective," *Global Public Health* 8, no. 1 (2013): 55–64.

208. "Research indicates risks of consuming high fructose corn syrup," University of Oxford, accessed July 17, 2013, http://www.ox.ac.uk/media/news_stories/2012/121128.html.

209. R. H. Lustig, "Fructose: it's 'alcohol without the buzz,'" *Advanced Nutrition* 4, no. 2 (2013): 226–235.

210. G. A. Bray and B. M. Popkin, "Calorie-sweetened beverages and fructose: what have we learned 10 years later," *Pediatric Obesity* 8, no. 4 (2013): 242–248.

211. G. A. Bray, "Energy and fructose from beverages sweetened with sugar or high-fructose corn syrup pose a health risk for some people," *Advanced Nutrition* 4, no. 2 (2013): 220–225.

212. K. A. Page, et al., "Effects of fructose vs glucose on regional cerebral blood flow in brain regions involved with appetite and reward pathways," *JAMA* 309, no. 1 (2013): 63–70.

213. A. N. Payne, C. Chassard, and C. Lacroix, "Gut microbial adaptation to dietary consumption of fructose, artificial sweeteners and sugar alcohols: implications for host-microbe interactions contributing to obesity," *Obesity Reviews* 13, no. 9 (2012): 799–809.

214. M. Basaranoglu, et al., "Fructose as a key player in the development of fatty liver disease," *World Journal of Gastroenterology* 19, no. 8 (2013): 1166–1172.

215. R. E. Morgan, "Does consumption of high-fructose corn syrup beverages cause obesity in children?" *Pediatric Obesity* 8, no. 4 (2013): 249–254.

216. G. L. Blackburn, et al., "The effect of aspartame as part of a multidisciplinary weight-control program on short- and long-term control of body weight," *American Journal of Clinical Nutrition* 65, no. 2 (1997): 409–418.

217. W. Nseir, F. Nassar, and N. Assy, "Soft drinks consumption and nonalcoholic fatty liver disease," *World Journal of Gastroenterology* 16, no. 21 (2010): 2579–2588.

218. Q. Yang, "Gain weight by 'going diet?' Artificial sweeteners and the neurobiology of sugar cravings," *Yale Journal of Biology and Medicine* 83, no. 2 (2010): 101–108.

219. C. Fitch and K. S. Keim, "Position of the Academy of Nutrition and Dietetics: use of nutritive and nonnutritive sweeteners," *Journal of the Academy of Nutrition and Dietetics* 112, no. 5 (2012): 739–758.

220. H. E. Ford, et al., "Effects of oral ingestion of sucralose on gut hormone response and appetite in healthy normal-weight subjects," *European Journal of Clinical Nutrition* 65, no. 4 (2011): 508–513.

221. M. B. Abou-donia, et al., "Splenda alters gut microflora and increases intestinal p-glycoprotein and cytochrome p-450 in male rats," *Journal of Toxicology and Environmental Health* 71, no. 21 (2008): 1415–1429.

222. "Nutrition and healthy eating: Artificial sweeteners and other sugar substitutes," Mayo Clinic, accessed July 17, 2013, http://www.mayoclinic.com/health/artificial-sweeteners/MY00073/NSECTIONGROUP=2.

223. Ben Tinker, "Coca-Cola weighs in on obesity fight," *CNN Health*, January 16, 2013, accessed July 16, 2013, http://www.cnn.com/2013/01/14/health/coke-obesity.

224. A. L. Beck, et al., "Association of beverage consumption with obesity in Mexican American children," *Public Health Nutrition* 17, no. 2 (2013): 338–344.

225. S. Vasanti, et al., "Sugar-sweetened beverages and weight gain in children and adults: a systematic review and meta-analysis," *American Journal of Clinical Nutrition* 98, no. 4 (2013): 1084–1102, http://ajcn.nutrition.org/content/98/4/1084.full.pdf+html.

226. G. Lasater, C. Piernas, and B. M. Popkin, "Beverage patterns and trends among school-aged children in the US, 1989–2008," *Nutrition Journal* 10 (2011), http://www.ncbi.nlm.nih.gov/pmc/articles/PMC3196913/.

227. M. Maersk, et al., Sucrose-sweetened beverages increase fat storage in the liver, muscle, and visceral fat depot: a 6-mo randomized intervention study," *American Journal of Clinical Nutrition* 95, no. 2 (2012): 283–289.

228. L. I. Lesser, F. J. Zimmerman, D. A. Cohen, "Outdoor advertising, obesity, and soda consumption: a cross-sectional study," *BMC Public Health* 13, no. 1 (2013): 20.

229. Jon Entine, "Is 2013 a Watershed Year for the Anti-Obesity Movement?" *Forbes* November 29, 2012, accessed July 16, 2013, http://www.forbes.com/sites/jonentine/2012/11/29/is-2013-a-watershed-year-for-the-anti-obesity-movement/2/.

230. G. Fagherazzi, et al., "Consumption of artificially and sugar-sweetened beverages and incident type 2 diabetes in the Etude Epidemiologique aupres des femmes de la Mutuelle Generale de l'Education Nationale-European Prospective Investigation into Cancer and Nutrition cohort," *American Journal of Clinical Nutrition* 97, no. 3 (2013): 517–523.

231. M. Brooks, "Sweetened Drinks May Boost Depression, Coffee Reduce It," Medscape Website, accessed July 16, 2013, http://www.medscape.com/viewarticle/777356.

232. S. N. Bhupathiraju, "Changes in Coffee Intake and Subsequent Risk of Type 2 Diabetes: Three Large Cohorts of US Men and Women," *Diabetologia* 57, no. 7 (2014): 1346, http://www.ncbi.nlm.nih.gov/pmc/articles/PMC4115458/pdf/nihms593866.pdf.

233. L. A. Persad, "Energy drinks and the neurophysiological impact of caffeine," *Frontiers in Neuroscience* 5 (2011), http://www.ncbi.nlm.nih.gov/pmc/articles/PMC3198027/.

234. Leslie Pray, Ann L. Yaktine, and Diana Pankevich, *Caffeine in Food and Dietary Supplements: Examining Safety: Workshop Summary* (Washingon, DC: National Academies Press, 2014), http://www.ncbi.nlm.nih.gov/books/NBK202230/pdf/Bookshelf_NBK202230.pdf.

235. Y. Gu, S. Yu, and J. D. Lambert, "Dietary cocoa ameliorates obesity-related inflammation in high fat-fed mice," *European Journal of Nutrition* 53, no. 1 (2014): 149–158, doi:10.1007/s00394-013-0510-1.

236. M. C. Andújar, "Cocoa Polyphenols and Their Potential Benefits for Human Health," *Oxidative Medicine and Cellular Longevity*, (2012), http://www.hindawi.com/journals/omcl/2012/906252/.

237. W. Wu, et al., "Coffee consumption and bladder cancer: a meta-analysis of observational studies," *Scientific Reports*, 5 (2015), http://www.nature.com/srep/2015/150312/srep09051/full/srep09051.html.

238. R. S. Keast, et al., "The influence of caffeine on energy content of sugar-sweetened beverages: 'the caffeine-calorie effect,'" *European Journal of Clinical Nutrition* 65, no. 12 (2011): 1338–44.

239. A. Szpak, D. Allen, "A case of acute suicidality following excessive caffeine intake," *Journal of Psychopharmacology* (Oxford) 26, no. 11 (2012): 1502–1510.

240. M. M. Peña and E. M. Taveras, "Preventing childhood obesity: wake up, it's time for sleep!" *Journal of Clinical Sleep Medicine* 7, no. 4 (2011): 343–344.

241. M. B. Schneider and H. J. Benjamin, "Sports drinks and energy drinks for children and adolescents: are they appropriate?" *Pediatrics* 127, no. 6 (2011): 1182–1189.

242. S. E. Swithers, et al., "Body weight gain in rats consuming sweetened liquids. Effects of caffeine and diet composition," *Appetite* 55, no. 3 (2010): 528–533.

243. M. M. Manore, "Dietary supplements for improving body composition and reducing body weight: where is the evidence?" *International Journal of Sport Nutrition and Exercise Metabolism* 22 (2012): 139–154.

244. A. M. Arria and M. C. O'Brien, "The 'high' risk of energy drinks," *JAMA* 305, no. 6 (2011): 600–601.

CHAPTER 14

245. R. Chhabra, S. Kolli, J. H. Bauer, "Organically grown food provides health benefits to Drosophila melanogaster," *PLOS ONE* 8, no. 1 (2013):e52988.

246. "What is the meaning of 'natural' on the label of food?" FDA, accessed July 17, 2013, http://www.fda.gov/AboutFDA/Transparency/Basics/ucm214868.htm.

247. L. Crowley, "HFCS is natural, says FDA in a letter," *Food Navigator*, accessed July 17, 2013http://www.foodnavigator-usa.com/Suppliers2/HFCS-is-natural-says-FDA-in-a-letter.

248. C. Smith-spangler, et al., "Are organic foods safer or healthier than conventional alternatives?: a systematic review," *Annals of Internal Medicine* 157, no. 5 (2012): 348–366.

249. "The Organic Watergate—White Paper Connecting the Dots: Corporate Influence at the USDA's National Organic Program," Cornucopia Institute, accessed July 17, 2013, http://www.cornucopia.org/USDA/OrganicWatergateWhitePaper.pdf.

250. J. Levasseur and V. L. Kubinec, "Pesticide residue found on nearly half of organic produce," *CBC News*, accessed April 15, 2014, http://www.cbc.ca/news/canada/manitoba/pesticide-residue-found-on-nearly-half-of-organic-produce-1.2487712.

251. J. Krauss, I. Gallenberger, and I. Steffan-dewenter, "Decreased functional diversity and biological pest control in conventional compared to organic crop fields," *PLOS ONE* 6, no. 5 (2011): e19502.

252. See https://www.biodynamics.com/biodynamics.html (accessed July 17, 2013).

253. R. Spaccini, et al., "Molecular properties of a fermented manure preparation used as field spray in biodynamic agriculture," *Environmental Science and Pollution Research International* 19, no. 9 (2012): 4214–4225.

254. Derek Thompson, "How America Spends Money: 100 Years in the Life of the Family Budget," *The Atlantic*, April 5, 2012, accessed July 17, 2013, http://www.theatlantic.com/business/archive/2012/04/how-america-spends-money-100-years-in-the-life-of-the-family-budget/255475/.

255. See Genesis 5:5.

256. "WHO Global Health Expenditure Atlas," World Health Organization, accessed July 17, 2013, http://www.who.int/nha/atlas.pdf.

CHAPTER 15

257. A. Drewnowski, "Concept of a nutritious food: toward a nutrient density score," *The American Journal of Clinical Nutrition* 82, no. 4 (2005): 721–732.

258. F. S. Atkinson, K. Foster-Powell, and J. C. Brand-Miller, "International Tables of Glycemic Index and Glycemic Load Values: 2008," *Diabetes Care* 31, no. 12 (2008).

259. A. J. Meinders and A. E. Meinders, "How much water do we really need to drink?" *Nederlands Tijdschrift voor Geneeskunde* 154 (2010): A1757.

260. A. Pan, et al., "Changes in water and beverage intake and long-term weight changes: results from three prospective cohort studies," *International Journal of Obesity* 37, no. 10 (2013): 1378–1385, http://www.ncbi.nlm.nih.gov/pmc/articles/PMC3628978/pdf/nihms-428475.pdf.

261. B. M. Popkin, K. E. D'Anci, and I. H. Rosenberg, "Water, hydration and health," Nutrition Reviews 68, no. 8 (2010): 439–458.

262. M. Millard-Stafford, et al., "Thirst and hydration status in everyday life," *Nutrition Reviews* 70, no. 2 (2012): S147.

263. For more information, visit http://www.purative.com/2012/01/scientists-say-dont-be-duped-by-alkaline-water/.

264. R. Slovak, "Quality, healthful water matters-Now let's find it or will someone please point the way to healthful water?" *Public Health Alert* 7, no. 5 (2012): 1–2, 9, http://publichealthalert.org/uploads/2012_5.pdf.

265. Based on the Glycemic Index. For more helpful information on the Glycemic Index, visit http://www.glycemicindex.com (accessed April 15, 2014).

266. "All 48 Fruits and Vegetables with Pesticide Residue Data," Environmental Working Group, accessed April 15, 2014, http://www.ewg.org/foodnews/list.php.

267. J. Perez-Jimenez, V. Neveu, and A. Scalbert, "Identification of the 100 richest dietary sources of polyphenols: an application of the Phenol-Explorer database," *European Journal of Clinical Nutrition* 64 (2010): S112–120.

268. M. H. Carlsen, et al., "The total antioxidant content of more than 3100 foods, beverages, spices, herbs and supplements used worldwide," *Nutrition Journal* 9, no. 3 (2010): 1–11.

269. Based on the Glycemic Index and the ANDI Food Score. For more information on the Glycemic Index, visit http://www.glycemicindex.com, and for more information on the ANDI Food Score, a system created by Dr. Furhman which rates nutrition, visit http://www.drfuhrman.com.

270. For another helpful source that features an ANDI Guide, visit http://www.wholefoodsmarket.com. For more information on comparative pesticide residue levels, see http://www.ncbi.nlm.nih.gov/pmc/articles/PMC3297498/pdf/1744-8603-8-2.pdf.

271. J. Perez-Jimenez, V. Neveu, and A. Scalbert, "Identification of the 100 richest dietary sources of polyphenols: an application of the Phenol-Explorer database," *European Journal of Clinical Nutrition* 64 (2010): S112–120.

272. S. M. Chacko, et al., "Beneficial effects of green tea: A literature review," *Chinese Medicine* 5, no. 13 (2010): 1–6. For more information on the health benefits of green tea, visit http://umm.edu/health/medical/altmed/herb/green-tea.

273. Based on the ANDI Food Score. For more information on the ANDI Food Score, a system created by Dr. Furhman which rates nutrition, visit http://www.drfuhrman.com.

274. J. Perez-Jimenez, V. Neveu, and A. Scalbert, "Identification of the 100 richest dietary sources of polyphenols: an application of the Phenol-Explorer database," *European Journal of Clinical Nutrition* 64 (2010): S112–120.

275. Based on the Glycemic Index. For more helpful information on the Glycemic Index, visit http://www.glycemicindex.com (accessed April 15, 2014).

276. Based on the ANDI Food Score. For more information on the ANDI Food Score, a system created by Dr. Furhman which rates nutrition, visit http://www.drfuhrman.com.

277. J. Perez-Jimenez, V. Neveu, and A. Scalbert, "Identification of the 100 richest dietary sources of polyphenols: an application of the Phenol-Explorer database," *European Journal of Clinical Nutrition* 64 (2010): S112–120.

278. See http://www.ncbi.nlm.nih.gov/pmc/articles/PMC3981995/.

279. P. Chan, et al., "A double-blind placebo-controlled study of the effectiveness and tolerability of oral stevioside in human hypertension," *British Journal of Clinical Pharmacology* 50, no. 3 (2000): 215–220.

CHAPTER 17

280. R. R. Wing and S. Phelan, "Long-term weight loss maintenance," *American Journal of Clinical Nutrition* 82, no. 1 (2005): 222S–2225S.

281. "Top Four Reasons Why Diets Fail," *Science Daily*, accessed July 17, 2013, http://www.sciencedaily.com/releases/2013/01/130103192352.htm.

282. L. Bacon, et al., "Size acceptance and intuitive eating improve health for obese, female chronic dieters," *Journal of the American Dietetic Association* 105, no. 6 (2005): 929–936.

283. L. E. Burke, J. Wang, and M. A. Sevick, "Self-monitoring in weight loss: A systematic review of the literature," *Journal of the American Dietetic Association* 111, no. 1 (2011): 92–102.

284. B. Fjedsoe, et al., "'Get Healthy, Stay Healthy': protocol for evaluation of a lifestyle intervention delivered by text-message following the Get Healthy Information and Coaching Service®," *BMC Public Health* 14, no. 112 (2014).

285. C. Dellasega, R. M. Anel-Tiangco, and R. A. Gabbay, "How patients with type 2 Diabetes Mellitus respond to motivational interviewing," *Diabetes Research and Clinical Practice* 95, no. 1 (2012): 37–41.

286. S. Rubak, et al., "Motivational interviewing: a systematic review and meta-analysis," *British Journal of General Practice* 55, no. 513 (2005): 305–312.

287. L. A. Simmons and R. Q. Wolever, "Integrative health coaching and motivational interviewing: Synergistic approaches to behavior change in healthcare," *Global Advances in Health and Medicine* 2, no. 4 (2013): 28.

288. P. Ryan, "Integrated theory of health behavior change," *Clinical Nurse Specialist* 23, no. 3 (2009): 161–72.

289. P. J. Teixeira, et al., "Motivation, self-determination, and long-term weight control," *International Journal of Behavioral Nutrition and Physical Activity* 9, no. 22 (2012): 1–13.

290. C. Duhigg, *The Power of Habit, Why We Do What We Do in Life and Business* (New York: Random House, 2012).

291. T. M. Leahey and R. R. Wing, "A randomized controlled pilot study testing three types of health coaches for obesity treatment: professional, peer, and mentor," *Obesity* 21, no. 5 (2013): 1–8.

292. J. H. Rimmer, et al., "Telehealth weight management intervention for adults with physical disabilities: a randomized controlled trial," *American Journal of Physical and Medical Rehabilitation* 92, no. 12 (2013): 1084.

293. K. O. Hwang, et al., "Social support in an Internet weight loss community," *International Journal of Medical Informatics* 79, no. 1 (2010): 5–13.

CHAPTER 18

294. B. Gardner, "Making health habitual: the psychology of 'habit-formation' and general practice," *British Journal of General Practice* 62, no. 605 (2012): 664–666.

295. R. J. Beeken, et al., "Study protocol for the 10 Top Tips (10TT) trial: Randomised controlled trial of habit-based advice for weight control in general practice," *BMC Public Health* 2, no. 12 (2012): 667.

296. J. O. Hill, "Can a small-changes approach help address the obesity epidemic? A report of the Joint Task Force of the American Society for Nutrition, Institute of Food Technologist, and International Food Information Council," *American Journal of Clinical Nutrition* 89, no. 2 (2009): 477–484.

297. See 3 John 2.

INDEX

ABOUT THE AUTHOR

David Nico, "Dr. Healthnut," is a certified wellness coach who helps leaders live well so they can model vitality, inspire vision, and create legacy. He's like a one-stop-doc for well-being. *Diet Diagnosis* is his first book in the Dr. Healthnut series, which is a comprehensive guide on truly nourishing your body. Please connect with him at drhealthnut.com, @drhealthnut on Twitter, and at facebook.com/drhealthnut.

HEALTHNUT LIFE WEEK ___

Step #1: Remember my Healthnut Inspire (see page 203)

Step #2: My Healthnut *Aha!* (see page 205)

My Healthnut Awareness:

_____

_____

_____

My Healthnut Hopes and Actions (rate Actions on 1–5 scale):

Hope #1: I will _____

_____.

    Action: This week, I'll _____

_____.[ ]

Hope #2: I will _____

_____.

    Action: This week, I'll _____

_____.[ ]

Hope #3: I will _____

_____.

    Action: This week, I'll _____

_____.[ ]

Hope #4: I will _____

_____.

    Action: This week, I'll _____

_____.[ ]

HOPE #5: I will _____

_____.

    Action: This week, I'll _____

_____.[   ]

HOPE #6: I will _____

_____.

    Action: This week, I'll _____

_____.[   ]

Step #3: My Healthnut Fans: Week ____ Appointments

1. _____

_____

2. _____

_____

3. _____

_____

Healthnut Score Week ___: _____

HEALTHNUT LIFE WEEK ___

Step #1: Remember my Healthnut Inspire (see page 203)

Step #2: My Healthnut *Aha!* (see page 205)

My Healthnut Awareness:

_____

_____

_____

My Healthnut Hopes and Actions (rate Actions on 1–5 scale):

HOPE #1: I will _____

_____.

   Action: This week, I'll _____

_____.[ ]

HOPE #2: I will _____

_____.

   Action: This week, I'll _____

_____.[ ]

HOPE #3: I will _____

_____.

   Action: This week, I'll _____

_____.[ ]

HOPE #4: I will _____

_____.

   Action: This week, I'll _____

_____.[ ]

Hope #5: I will _____

_____.

    Action: This week, I'll _____

_____.[ ]

Hope #6: I will _____

_____.

    Action: This week, I'll _____

_____.[ ]

Step #3: My Healthnut Fans: Week ____ Appointments

1. _____

_____

2. _____

_____

3. _____

_____

Healthnut Score Week ____: _____